MAGNIFICENT MISERY
From Adversity to Ecstasy

For more information, go to:
https://www.yourmagnificencementor.com

Paperback Second Edition: October 2022
First Digital Edition: October 2022

Cover design by: Jack Born, Design Quarry

Published by:

FingerTip Solutions – Edmonton, Alberta,
and
Legacy Lane Publishing
Weatherford, TX
www.LegacyLanePublishing.com

ISBN 979-8-224-61916-0 (paperback – second edition)
ISBN 978-1-894393-03-4 (digital)

Dear Chantel,

How lovely we're on
this magnificent
journey together

Bless You!

Sera

What Readers are saying about Magnificent Misery:

"Magnificent Misery" will resonate with anyone who has ever gone through a serious health challenge. When death looked Sue in the eye, she evoked a little humor to soothe the raw edges of this amazing story of strength and courage. So real, so open, and such a gift to the reader.

Dianna Bowes, Founder of Fabulous@50

Magnificent Misery is must-read; an eloquent balance of inspiration, enlightenment, and entertainment expressed through a real-life story. Sue has a way of pulling you into her experiences; you feel you're right there with her – not only enduring her trials and tribulations, but also reaping the priceless wisdom she acquired because of them. I wanted to leap into the pages to hold her hand as she stomached and inevitably overcame seemingly insurmountable obstacles. Ironically, it is her story that will hold the hand of anyone going through any hardship because one way or another, her story is our story.

Dan King, Soul Coach, Speaker & Author of SOULgasm Series

I started your book before bed...AND COULDN'T STOP UNTIL I FINISHED IT! I kept telling myself, "Only one more chapter"...nope, never happened because your book was too compelling. The flow of your personal story took me on a roller coaster...I was smiling with you, crying with you, rooting for you...

I finally went to bed with a head full of new, insightful, hopeful thoughts about myself and the world/universe. Thank you, Miss Sue.

Meesha Lee

Never could I have imagined the impact of the book by Sue Paulson. Her book took me on a phenomenal journey of one magnificent woman. Sue's candid, raw, and vibrant energy has caused a huge ripple in me! She has opened up an untouched part of my Soul and given me an incredible number of gifts in return for reading "Magnificent Misery".

Tonya Alton, Author

Sue's description of her journey is a deep, intimate study of the soul and heart of somebody going through the experience. She shares her fears and struggle inherent in making the right decisions on her journey toward health and healing.

After meditating about the many ideas contained in the book, I realized that it was a practitioner's dream, for we always struggle to obtain from our clients a critical and productive perspective on the meaning of a sickness.

Cancer is an opportunity for the client to re-engineer his/her life. It is an opportunity for transformation; Sue clearly achieved this transformation.

Francisco Valenzuela
MA.DCH.PhD. Author *Psycho-Oncology, Hypnosis and Psychosomatic Healing in Cancer*

Your book astonished me, Sue. Such a dauntlessly wise and compassionate spirit you are! You exposed me to the feathered edges of just how large a human being can grow.

Teri Ebel

Dedication

This book is dedicated to all who have faced, are facing, or who will face adversity. Even though it may feel like it – you are not alone. Bless you for your courage in facing your trials and tribulations for your highest good and the good of all on Planet Earth. If you choose it, ecstasy awaits just
on the other side of
any misery - I
promise!

Acknowledgements

Just as "no man is an island", a writer never births a book without help. I tip my hat to Jack Born of Design Quarry for a beautiful cover and to Rob at Rob Merkel Designs for initial content formatting. Diane Bell of Legacy Lane Publishing has been invaluable in launching this second edition.

To my original manuscript readers: Andrea Collins, Carla Janzen, Dan King, Cathy Mercredi, and Dr. Francisco Valenzuela – your feedback was so helpful. To the U of A Writer in Residence, Minister (Malcolm) Faust – not only were your comments very encouraging, but your great advice also made a difference during the revision process.

Blessings to paramedics, Dan and Eric and to Dr. Baydock and all the medical staff at Grey Nuns who saved my life in 2007.

Dr. Nawaid Usmani, my oncologist, the Cross Cancer team, and surgeon, Dr. Erica Haase from Grey Nun's demonstrated their compassion and skills throughout treatment and recovery. My dear friend, Ta-ee-a Bryce eased the pain of a difficult hospital stay.

Naturopath, Dr. DeNault of Optimum Wellness helped promote a return to full health, while Dr. Francisco Valenzuela, Hypnotherapist, Psychologist, Dr. Matilde Valenzuela worked gently and diligently to help free me from my prison of destructive beliefs.

It was on the shores of Kardamyli in Greece where I pulled my manuscript together, thanks to writing coach and intrepid guide, Suzanne Harris. Elias and Mrs. Antonia, our hosts, welcomed us with open arms and encouraged us in our work.

Finally, to my dear friends and family, I'm very grateful for all your love and support as I journey through this lifetime. It's an honor to have you by my side.

Note from the Author

My Grammy Ed used to say, "Well, I don't want to miss out on anything in this life." Over the course of her 87 years, she didn't miss much. I seem to be following in her footsteps.

A curious sort of person, I've always wanted to know the whys and how's of many things – especially those that impacted my life and helped me to grow as a person.

It's been said that *truth is stranger than fiction.* I would agree wholeheartedly. No fiction I've ever read quite matches the wildness of the rollercoaster ride that I've experienced in this lifetime.

Vastly different from my previous *how to* books, this book is a memoir. It documents eight of the most significant years of my life, along with brief forays into my early history to provide some context. Some of the names of individuals involved have been changed to protect their privacy.

Because of the extremely personal nature of my journey, I questioned my reasons for making it public. I also wondered whether it mattered at all if I told my story. Elias Polimeneas, a very wise philosopher and Greek poet said to me: *"Your story is not just your story – it's our story. It matters to us."*

I have taken his advice with the hope that you, my reader, will benefit in some way from my sharing. As I close that chapter of my life with this book, I hold the lessons and gifts from that time close to my heart. From here, it's onward and upward to the next grand adventure – for all of us!

Table of Contents

*Amidst passion, the
Specter of Death came
knocking.*

*It was a balmy Saturday
night, that
July in
2007.*

*How bizarre that in one
instant, a person could move
from "dying to have sex" to
dying from having sex.*

*Even stranger is my story
of how that event led to
the spiritual path of
full-blown ecstasy...*

Sue Paulson

Chapter 1

There are some things you learn best in calm, some in storm.

Willa Cather

I am 57 – single again after a second marriage of 23 years had ended. Like many marriages, it had its ups and downs, its struggles, and triumphs. In the early days, we had worked hard on our relationship to resolve conflicts and differences. As our son got older, my husband and I drifted apart, until the loneliness I felt inside the marriage became too much to bear. Painful though it was to leave, it was even harder to stay.

Four years as a single woman has sped by. I've been blessed with an amazing son, have experienced success as a speaker and self-published author, and I am engaged in meaningful work. Despite my full new life, I am lonely. I begin to wonder if there might be a "third time lucky" partner for me. Not only am I afraid of living the rest of my days as a dried-up old divorcee with six cats for company, but I've also begun to feel those almost forgotten urges to connect with a man. Horny hormones start to emerge.

Quite frankly, aside from wanting to find my soul mate, I am dying to have sex – though I'm embarrassed to admit that out loud! I'd quipped to a close friend recently, "I want to experience full-blown ecstasy before I die." All the heroines in romance novels seem to achieve sexual ecstasy. Why not me?

But the idea of dating again is scary – first, I fret about who would want me at my age. The reality of dating in 2007 is not the way it had been in my 20s. I do not travel in circles filled with eligible men, nor do my married friends know any eligible singles. All my available girlfriends are struggling to find partners, too.

My younger friends keep prodding me to try online dating. Even though the notion of it does not thrill me, I am afraid of missing out; it seems to be my only hope. So, I get as much advice as I can from those in the know, have my picture taken, write my profile, and venture online.

Lavalife is the first site I cruise through. Dating sites have not been around that long. Some I find very difficult to navigate, plus I have this aversion to paying to connect with someone. I spend the grand sum of $18.00 for my first round of contact credits.

Connecting with potential dates online is very much a sorting process. Most guys have skimpy profiles and little to say for themselves, so it is hard to strike up a screen conversation. Then there are those who are long on promise and short on delivery. Much like a hyped-up resume, someone might showcase nicely online, but the first telephone chat reveals a Jekyll & Hyde split.

My adventures become the source of eager conversation amongst my buddies who are too chicken to go online themselves. Believe me, I soon have plenty of bad but amusing stories to share - a writer's dream come true!

After a few unproductive coffee dates and one disastrous offline encounter with a man from church, I find a fellow – Mark - who makes it very clear in his profile that "chemistry" is the main reason he is dating. His picture is nice, and he seems to be able to describe himself without spelling mistakes or poor grammar. Hmmm - until Mr. Right comes along, maybe some sexual release will work nicely. Guilt pokes at me – old puritan programming – good grief! Can't I have some fun?

A few e-mails lead to phone calls. We meet for the first time at a local driving range. Mark is waiting for me as I pull my clubs out of the car. He is about 5' 8'', slim, and pleasant looking. We chat between shots – it had been so long since I'd dated, that I didn't notice him admiring my form – I thought he was checking out my golf swing! At 53, Mark has familiar, old-fashioned manners. He opens doors, helps me with my coat, compliments me on my looks, and buys me dinner.

A couple of dates and a few kisses later signals chemistry to be alive and raring to go. We eventually reveal our respective pink parts to each other.

Now if you're a post-menopausal woman reading this, you may know that as we age, juicy ideas in bed don't always match with our aging vagina's ability. Maybe you, like me have already experienced the vaginal dryness that accompanies declining hormones. My family doctor had already indicated that I had some vaginal atrophy. I know it's important to have a sensitive, considerate, and patient lover.

Mark and I have a frank discussion. I tell him it has been a while since I've had intercourse and that dryness is a concern. We agree to take it slow. I buy lubricant. He proves to be a skilled and imaginative lover and treats me with care and consideration. Over time, our sessions become more intense, but intercourse is still painful.

One fateful day in July 2007, when I ask to stop a more vigorous love- making session, I go from *dying to have sex* to dying from *having* sex. Unbeknownst to us, we have lacerated an artery high in my vaginal wall. I don't feel much pain, but Mark asks if I am bleeding, so I check myself in the bathroom.

The toilet fills with blood more than once. Hoping it will stop, I shower off and diaper myself in a towel. I cuddle in Mark's arms with my feet propped up on the wall. Will the bleeding stop?

I think about going to hospital. His offer to drive worries me. What about the long wait in Emergency? What if I soak his car seat? "Do you have ambulance coverage?" he asks. I struggled to decide - what to wear, how to manage. I have no sanitary supplies. My concentration wavers as I start to feel woozy and disoriented.

"Call 911 - I need the ambulance." Mark calls and briefly describes the situation. They arrive quickly. I hear them ask at the door, "Is it your mother?" I can hear the discomfort in Mark's voice as he says no. How embarrassing!

Then two paramedics, young enough to be my sons, enter my bedroom. Embarrassment number two - to have to confess the reason for my predicament. Bless these two professionals who don't bat an eye as I relate the bald truth of my situation.

Dressed only in a large, dark towel, my tee shirt, and socks, I am wrapped discreetly into blankets, strapped to the stretcher, and rolled to the waiting ambulance. Mark agrees to lock up and meet me at Emergency. Dan and Eric wait for directions from headquarters as I am prepped for an IV drip and have my blood pressure recorded.

A bustling Saturday night, my two rescuers seem grateful to have a "normal" person to transport instead of the usual challenges from barroom brawls and overdoses. We chat and joke on the bumpy ride to the hospital. An ambulance ride is not comfortable!

Emergency is busy, with empty ambulances parked bumper to bumper as the EMTs wait to transfer patients to hospital staff. I begin to feel nauseous and weak. Eric signals Dan, who wheels an oxygen tank over, tucks the prongs in my nose and hooks me up to an IV drip. Despite the continuous internal pulse of the bleeding, I start to feel better. The nurse comes by to assure me of help in just a little bit.

Finally, a room is available. Blood has started to soak through to the top of the blankets. I worry about all the bedclothes I am soiling and wonder how they will transfer me from the stretcher. I don't want those nice young men to see all the mess I've made. I needn't have worried. First, they strip the bed I am moving to, and then easily transfer me, blankets and all, with no fuss or loss of my dignity. Phew!

Linda introduces herself as my nurse - my age or perhaps a bit older. She is kindness personified. Her calm and matter of fact approach soothes me. I tell her my story. Once she has me settled, she finds Mark in the waiting room and ushers him in.

"How are you doing?" he asks. I assure him I am in good hands and ask if he'd go back to my apartment for my cell phone, my day planner, and the clothes I'd forgotten to bring. He promises to return as soon as he can – what a way to end a date!

The young emergency resident arrives - are they all this young? He appears unflappable as he examines me internally.

Of course, a pelvic exam avoided a few months ago due to extreme discomfort at my doctor's is now a necessity. At the click of the speculum expanding, the pain is beyond intense. Hearing my sharp intake of breath, Linda asks if I am OK. Though I feel like screaming, I do my best to breathe through the pain. Decades of lessons in "how to behave properly in public" kick in. I don't make a fuss, even though I want to.

The doctor locates the source of the bleed and then calls for the resident gynecologist. Young and bright, her manner is soothing and gentle. She talks me through the second pelvic exam. More painful than the first, I stay as still as I can, though they might have to scrape me from the ceiling. Linda comments on how well I am doing. "You're very stoic," she says.

We discuss my two options - pack the area and hope the bleeding stops or go into surgery to stitch up the lacerated artery. Since I've already lost so much blood, there is only one decision. I am relieved to hear that they will put me under while they repair the damage. Linda is pleasantly surprised when she hears that it will only be another 30 minutes before the operation.

Mark arrives with my stuff. Bless his heart, he'd taken time to strip the bedding and left it in the tub to soak. Though he wants to stay, I tell him to go home. "I'll call tomorrow when I'm out of surgery."

I bask in the support I receive as I am moved to surgery. I feel a well of gratitude for these competent, caring souls who work so diligently in the middle of the night. I tell them what a great team I have.

As I wait for the anesthetic, I marvel that I am not in pain. Maybe I'm too scared to even feel scared, so I deny the fear and just deal with the moments before me. I think about dying. This could be it. My thoughts flit to my son. How will he cope if I don't make it? A flash of regret fills me as they wheel me into surgery.

I wake up in recovery, groggy, struggling to talk - to let the staff know I am okay. My recovery nurse is sweet, helpful. I fade in and out, and then find myself on the hospital ward, bed 4203B. It is early Sunday morning. Dr. Baydock, my surgeon drops by. All I remember about her visit is her instruction to book an appointment in four to six weeks.

By mid-afternoon, I start thinking again of my son who has been away camping with his girlfriend. I dread making the phone call - seriously consider not telling him at all. It would spare us both some agony. One part of me desperately needs the support of family and friends; the other part is loath to admit what has just happened.

I am afraid of being judged, or worse, pitied. Growing up, I was clueless about my sexuality – in fact the subject was taboo in our household. And sexuality at my age – outrageous (or so I believed). It is not my nature to tell lies, yet I struggle to find the words for the unvarnished truth, especially when feeling so vulnerable.

I call Trevor and just tell him I am in hospital but am fine. I can hear the worry in his voice, especially when I don't share any details. While I wait for my son, I phone my friend, Joy in Calgary. She is horrified, supportive, and amused, all at the same time. I feel so blessed to have her continued love and understanding.

Mark shows up full of concern. I assure him I am fine and will connect once I am home from the hospital. I keep the visit short because I don't want him here when Trevor shows up.

Trevor and his girlfriend, Kristina arrived soon after. I marvel at his calm acceptance as I tell them, face to face, what I've been up to. Since I have no control over what they might think or feel about this situation, I state it as simply as if I'd cut my finger making a peanut butter sandwich. These poor kids - life gets a bit raw sometimes.

Chapter 2

The wound is the place where the light enters you. **Rumi**

With plenty of time to just "be" while coping with recovery in hospital, awareness dawns that my brush with death had transported me to the Afterlife – Heaven – the Great Beyond. I don't remember "going to the Light", as I have read about in other near-death experiences. Nor do I remember meeting anyone or having my past roll in front of me, like a movie screen.

Instead, it was both a knowing and a full body feeling. For a time, I basked in this remarkable place where I reveled in the bliss and joy of Oneness –truly experiencing full-blown, spiritual ecstasy.

Picture yourself floating in a vast sea of Unconditional Love and acceptance – embraced and supported in all ways simply and especially because you are an integral, essential, and magnificent part of all that is – Spirit, God, the Universe – whatever name fits for you.

That's what I experienced. There was nothing I had to **do** to claim my spot except remember that this is where I belong. Best of all, there was no fear – I felt safe.

I experienced the divine perfection of all that is. In the grand scheme of the Universe, no one thing, person, or idea matters any more than the next. All are integral parts of the whole. It all matters, yet none of it matters.

The most surprising revelation - judgment in this realm does not exist. There is no book, no day of reckoning to compare my "good deeds" with my "bad deeds". Polarities – right-wrong, good-bad – don't exist, either. Saint or sinner – all are equal – none better than another. Everything that happens on earth is unfolding, growing, and evolving as is meant to.

This bliss, this taste of spiritual ecstasy is powerful beyond belief. I know now from that experience that death as we believe it to be is merely an illusion. We all are everlasting, spiritual beings having a human experience. Our ideas of dying might be horrible, but death itself is nothing to fear. Although we do leave our earthly bodies by "dying", our Spirit lives on, for we are eternal Beings.

Amidst the memory of all that bliss, my physical reality intrudes. By Monday, I am feeling well enough for my first shower. Oh, the bliss of water streaming over my body! Gazing in the bathroom mirror as I dry off, I notice how very pale my face is. When the resident drops by, she asks if I feel ready to go home. I request that she test my blood.

"I'm not usually so pale," I say. One test and two hours later, a couple of bags of blood are hooked up to my I.V. I guess I was down a quart!

As they pick me up from hospital on Tuesday, my kids fuss round me like mother hens. They beg to take me home with them for a couple days, but all I want is my own bed and the peace of my apartment. They promise to bring me food – I promise to rest.

I make a few calls to friends and one to Kevin, my chiropractor, to book an appointment. When I arrive at his office a couple days later, he asks what has happened. "You've been on my mind since Sunday," he says. "I knew something dramatic must have been going on."

A skilled energy worker who has helped me through many transitions in the 12 years I have known him; he works his usual magic and suggests I book another visit soon.

On Saturday night, at my invitation, Mark drops by with a pizza. "Look", I said. "I don't want you to feel guilty about what happened. It's not your fault. I'm going to be just fine." We talk about his week, and I thank him for all his support through my ordeal. His chaste, goodbye kiss signals a definite shift in our relationship.

Sunday finds me on the golf course at the invitation of my friend, Suzie. Her mother-in-law, an avid golfer at 87, is in town visiting. Knowing how much I liked to golf, Suzie urges me to join the foursome.

Always at peace on the golf course, I marvel anew at the vibrant greens, the jeweled flowers, fresh, clean air, and the beauty of nature. All my senses have been heightened since my brush with death. I am in awe of the life around me. I have a decent game, too, though the exertion exhausts me physically.

"What were you thinking?" asks Kevin the next day as he scolds me for being on the golf course so soon after surgery. "What happened to you is big. Your bladder meridian has reversed itself. This is serious!"

I meekly promise to smarten up and take better care of myself.

Journal - Early August

It's been an uphill battle to cope with a slower than expected physical recovery. Even worse is the emotional aftermath. Back on planet Earth, the peace and the euphoria I felt in Heaven is gone.

I'm angry at being sent back. Why couldn't I stay? Why show me the wonders of the Universe, and then push me out? I had this incredible experience, only to have the door slammed shut in my face. Did I not measure up? Was there some secret tally card – some test I failed?

Even worse, I seem to have lost my sense of purpose. If nothing matters to the Universe, then were all my efforts to find meaning and purpose wasted? I struggled for so many years to do and be good – to help others – to earn my ticket to Heaven. But if saints are no better than sinners, then was it pointless? I feel lost - I even feel like giving up. Nothing seems to matter. Part of me wonders who I am now. The other part of me has ceased to care.

For a week, I hang out in denial about the magnitude of the turmoil inside. As the pressure builds, another visit to Kevin sparks the catalyst to help me face the wellspring of emotion I have been avoiding. I spend the weekend weeping and grieving.

I start living life on different levels all at the same time. While very little seems to matter right now, on another level, I no longer take any sense of well- being for granted. I feel more grateful and more compassionate than ever before.

Doubts and questions compete with the beauty of the sun on my face. Green grass is as precious as the bright blue sky. My reverence for all life increases even as my despair grows. I share with my friend, Suzy my thoughts of going back, of ending it all.

"Sue, it's not that easy to intentionally check out." Of course, she's right. I resign myself to muddling through as best I can.

Life continues while I ride my emotional rollercoaster; a new job helps steer my mind away from frustrated internal musings. I bless work skills that kick in like cruise control.

Outwardly it appears as if I have my act together. My "could care less" attitude only surfaces in private moments. I mourn my former go-getter self. The myth about the phoenix rising from the ashes comes to mind, but all I feel are ashes, with nary a feather in sight.

It's September. I meet with Dr. Baydock, my surgeon/gynecologist whose specialty is women's health. For the dreaded pelvic exam, she assures me she will use the slimmest speculum possible. She is gentle and efficient. It still hurts. There is a bit more bleeding. Not usually squeamish, I flinch at the sight of it.

She pronounces me healed from the surgery – the good news. The bad news – I have a very severe case of atrophy for a woman my age. In addition to tissue-thin and very brittle walls, my vagina has shrunk to the size of a slim, tapered candle.

She asks about my desire for a healthy sex life. "Well, I wasn't planning to give up sex, at least not until I 'm 90," I quip. "All right then," she says. "Here's what happens next."

She explains that full recovery is a two-stage process. We will start first with hormone replacement therapy. She tells me that in Canada, other than oral HRT, there were only three options: an estrogen ring, a dissolving tablet inserted vaginally, and estrogen cream. I am not big enough inside for the ring and the action of the tablet is too slow at this point, so she prescribes the cream and gives instructions about the regimen for the next three months. Once my vaginal tissue is plump and healthy again, I will move to the next stage.

"Now let's talk about stage two," says Dr. Baydock. "I'll be right back." She returns with a plain white box. Nested inside are six vaginal dilators. They ranged in size from slim to fat – not anatomically correct but close enough to spark the imagination. I struggle to keep the smirk off my face.

These medicinal dildos are designed to re-stretch the vaginal walls to allow for increasingly bigger accommodation. My eyes widen at the size of number six – Big Ben - oh my – a worthy goal! As I order the box, I imagine asking a future lover to show me his while I show him mine!

The reality of at least six months of daily vaginal therapy is a bit of a downer, brightened only by the doctor's assertion that any external pleasuring is fine – even recommended. Wow – permission from the doctor to masturbate! No second opinion needed on that issue.

I invite Mark for coffee. Our relationship has cooled to a kind of maiden aunt/concerned nephew status. I tell him about my upcoming treatment protocol that will last at least six months. Deep down, I know that continuing our relationship is not an option.

I gently send him on his way, with the hope that there will be no lasting trauma for him. I imagine his ad for a new partner. "Are you dying to have sex?"

Chapter 3

Stay close to anything that makes you feel alive.
Hafiz

My box of goodies causes much discussion among all my "over 50" girlfriends. Because of what has happened to me, most of them have concerns about their own vaginal health – could they be at risk, too? My younger women friends are quick to relate my story to their mothers as a warning to check in with their doctors.

Most of my friends also hunger to learn more about their sexuality as mid-life adults. Early sex education, if any, was sketchy at best. Some notions even proved to be wrong.

Suzy and I decide to host a Passion Party to check out the toys available to us. "Adult" education at its finest, we decide to have some fun while we learn. I request an older rep with enough life experience to answer our questions.

Much to our surprise, we have a full house for our party. Even my friends from Calgary drive down. Stacy, our rep, demonstrates lotions, oils, and potions. Individually, we make trips to the bathroom to sample a few. OH, MY!

Then she pulls out the toys. We watch with rapt attention as she explains the various gadgets. When she unveils her version of Big Ben, you could have heard a pin drop as she demonstrates the lights, bells, and whistles – okay, maybe you only whistle afterward! As "he" was passed around for inspection, we roar with laughter at the very idea of having that bad boy entertain us.

Everyone studies the catalogue with more intensity than a college final. Individual counseling is held discreetly in another room. In my one-on-one chat with Stacy, I share my recent history and resulting challenges. She finds just the right items for my needs. Eager chatter buzzes around the tea pot. "What did you order?" "Really?!" "Well, I thought I'd try…" Of course, a couple weeks after our purchases arrive, the phone lines sizzle as we check in regarding the success of our experimentation – "jackpot" is the enthusiastic response!

In the meantime, Mark's disappearance creates that all-too-familiar Saturday night void. Feeling like damaged goods, I am sad and bitter about how my life seems to be turning out. Still, I cling to any glimmer of hope. I go back online and troll through the Plenty of Fish internet waters for any likely candidates.

There is one profile that intrigues me. His profile is thorough, and he is very specific about his criteria for a partner. Thinking he won't likely respond; I send him a saucy note anyway.

Much to my surprise and delight, he does write back. We start exchanging both short and lengthy messages filled with humor and spice. Eventually we share our real names. I give David my phone number. Witty repartee on both ends of the phone line has me dancing like a teenager.

Within a few weeks, I feel ready to meet this man; I pick the place for our coffee date. It's October 1. Dressed in a smart business suit with a gorgeous tie, David looks very corporate and somewhat stern. I find out later that he was a bit disappointed about my high neckline -cleavage is important to guys!

We talk for three hours – well I talk – he listens! My plan had been to ask most of the questions and learn about him, but he proves to be more skilled at the art of questioning. It is both awkward and fun. When we go our separate ways, I hope I've made a good impression, but I couldn't get a feel for his interest in me. If he calls, great. If not…

He does call and asks me to dinner. It is time to wear something feminine and flirty. At dinner, David showers me with compliments.

He tells me I have a very sexy brain. I can't recall any other guy ever telling me that I am smart. I revel in being intensely female – I decide to buy sensuous garments with plunging necklines just for him.

Schooled by his mother to be the consummate gentleman, David opens my doors, seats me at dinner, and helps me with my coat. It takes some practice to set aside my independent streak and let him take charge. Our attraction for each other grows as we start to share hopes and dreams for the future.

While I have been in search of full-blown ecstasy with a life partner who will value a deep and meaningful relationship; he, too, is looking for that ideal mate. We are both determined not to settle for less than what we desire.

I share with him that I'd had a brush with death, though not the details of how it had occurred.

Thanksgiving 2007

Outside of my day-to-day life, I feel myself spiraling down into depression. I start to seek more help, though not through western medicine.

My California Mastermind buddies who are aware of many different healing modalities share the name of a healer in Vancouver. Unsure, I research other possibilities. Over time, I have learned to trust my intuition, so I wait for a sign to point me in the right direction.

Pathways to Vancouver open so easily that I know it's where I need to be. It's Thanksgiving weekend – I am amazed that not only is she home but is willing to see me. I have much to be thankful for.

Mahara Brenna, a healer and re-birthing specialist, welcomes me into her home for my private session. The walls are covered with pictures of saints and spiritual masters from all faiths.

I share my story and the resulting feelings. We talk about the impact of coming back to life after my near death. I have been so angry – feeling cheated out of that blissful peace that could have been mine permanently. I want to know who shut those pearly gates in my face and sent me back.

Mahara gently asserts that it was my Higher Self who drew me back, not some all-powerful jury voting yea or nay. Apparently, there is still a reason for me to be on planet Earth, though I can't imagine what it could be. She asks about my childhood, my position in my birth family.

As the pieces of the Sue puzzle are revealed, a plan for my re-birthing session emerges. She explains our respective roles and the process that she will guide me through.

Her treatment room has no chairs, only a large mattress on the floor covered with lush, jewel-toned blankets and pillows. Surrounding the mattress are crystal bowls of various sizes. She invites me to tuck in under the covers and get comfy. Mahara's soothing voice guides me to the starting point.

It is an amazing journey back to my four-year-old self. I'd abandoned her long ago because it had not felt safe to be that exuberant, carefree girl. As I breathe her into my heart space, I begin to feel a wholeness I had not known I'd been longing for these past 53 years.

The resonance of the crystal bowls fills the room and works its magic right to the core of me. How blessed I feel to be in this time and place with such an incredible gift of healing.

I long to stay in this energy forever, but home is calling. With no budget to stay over one more night, I head for the airport. Exhausted beyond measure from the intensity of the session, it takes every ounce of strength to board the plane home.

At cruising altitude, I stare out the window at glorious purple clouds laced with the setting sun. Tears fill my eyes. Flying, I feel close to God.

Healing

Dearest Spirit,
Touch these shriveled walls
with your sacred kisses.
Coax moisture and life
into fragile tissue.

Long have I punished this body
for carnal thoughts.
Felt guilty and dirty
when visions of sweaty sex
sent my trembling hands to
furtively pleasure parts of me
that religions decreed even Man must not
savor unless pro-creating.

My love for me
has withered through
abuse and neglect.
No more will I invite in
that barrenness or
allow the act of love
to tempt me to demise.

I long to feel
passion flowing into muscle.
The deep pulsing of ecstasy
sending mindless shivers
from head to toe.
When I'm whole again
with lush pink folds of welcoming skin
cradling healthy veins,
send me a lover
whose knowing, gentle touch
awakens me anew.

Grant us then the wisdom
to connect as never before.
In that timeless rhythm
that is man and woman joined
with You.

After a bit of recovery time, I call David to share some of my healing experience from my Vancouver trip. We'd had a couple of dates before my trip – precious time spent enjoying one another. With my attraction to him growing, I know the time will soon come to share the full story of my brush with death.

The next Saturday, he takes me to dinner. When he arrives with white roses, I am moved to tears. I know that I can no longer prolong my silence. He needs to know of my physical condition sooner rather than later.

Back at my place after dinner, we sit on my couch. I gather my courage and take a deep breath. "There's something I need to share with you," I say. "First of all, I'm very attracted to you in every way, physically, emotionally, mentally, and spiritually."

Then, embarrassed but determined, I stumble through my tale of a previous lover whose vigorous lovemaking had brought me to the brink of death, necessitating my subsequent surgery. I tell him I am still healing internally and am working toward the return of a fully functioning vagina. I outline the resulting limitations I currently have regarding sexual intimacy and share the doctor's prognosis for full recovery.

I brace myself for his response, fearful yet prepared to watch him walk out the door. David says, "That took great courage to tell me, didn't it?" I nod. "Look," he continued, "there are plenty of ways to make love besides intercourse."

His reassurance is music to my ears. Then he, too, shares an intimate story of his own that takes equal courage. I find myself in awe of the inner beauty of this intense male gracing my living room. He leaves me with no doubt about his attraction to me – all of me. I begin to hope that there is a way for us to work through my challenge.

Meanwhile, daily life beckons. At my core, I struggle to find a purpose, any purpose. I work at easy jobs that have little meaning but fill my time and pay the bills. I wonder if I will ever emerge from the dark cave I seem to be living in.

While browsing the shops one day, I find a stunning turquoise phoenix on a chain. Though I have little money to spare, I buy it as my symbol of hope to rise from the ashes one day. My other solace comes from meditating morning and night to Mahara's CD. It brings me such comfort to hear her soothing voice.

David continues to shower me with compliments and attention. Our relationship progresses to the bedroom. He proves to be a skilled and considerate lover. While I adore his touch, I am not as responsive as I'd hoped to be.

It's puzzling and frustrating for both of us. There is no question that the many taboos and old programs about sex I learned growing up had contributed to me repressing my sexual identity. I also struggle with my fears of never being able to make love in the time-honored way.

In the car one day, David initiates a conversation about sex. A little voice in my head starts screeching at me, "He's talking about sex, in broad daylight, right out loud!" I am embarrassed and uncomfortable, but it's a relief to explore the topic of sexuality with someone as open and comfortable with it as David.

Eager to remove our intimacy blockage, I decide to book another session with Mahara – this time to explore issues around my sexuality. The trip is easier. Since I know what to expect from her session, the work I'd committed to before leaving just happens. Strange how old stuff lurks in one's very tissues and causes problems without us being aware of it.

At home, I ask for the help and support I need to move forward sexually. David professes to be a very willing participant. I relax more into our lovemaking, and we achieve better results.

On the work front, I continued to struggle with my purpose. I find I have little desire to promote the many skills and talents I have accumulated. Past glories and accomplishments mean little.

All too often, I feel so much less than the powerful man at my side who has accomplished so much and is so focused. Some days it seems as if I have done nothing with my life, despite writing and producing two books and teaching for so many years both corporately and at the college level.

I doubt that I can ever measure up to David. He is such a direct beam of forceful energy, while I wander around aimlessly in dazed circles. I don't feel worthy of his regard; nevertheless, I gather up my courage to tell him that I am in love with him. As I suspected he might, he has trouble taking it in – one of the few times I've seen him speechless!

When December arrives, I can't seem to get too excited about Christmas. Friends I usually visit are going away. David will head to Colorado to be with family.

With a meal at my place, we celebrate before he leaves. Generous with beautifully wrapped gifts, he surprises me with a heartfelt card on which he wrote, I love you. I am so moved I choke right up. As we cuddle, he says, "I can no longer deny how I feel about you."

Chapter 4

We don't receive wisdom; we must discover it for ourselves after a journey that no one can take for us or spare us. **Marcel Proust**

Just as who we have been and who we are shape our relationships, so, too, do our relationships continue to shape us as individuals. Life with David proves to be turbulent. His passionate fire sign and my gentle water sign are often at odds. When we click, it's wonderful – when we clash, it feels horrible. It's the ultimate in roller coaster rides, disturbing one moment and exhilarating the next.

After 11 months of connection, separation, then re-connection, we feel there is enough love to make a partnership work. David invites me to move in. I am hesitant, but my feelings for him are so strong, I am determined to make it work. While it is true that opposites attract, the practicalities of building a "happily ever after" with said opposites would prove more daunting than either of us could anticipate.

In September 2008 I move in with him. He had recently bought a townhouse that is bigger than my apartment. However, because it is fully furnished, there is little room for any of my furniture, so I will sell or give most of mine away. Much to my surprise, I shed many tears over the loss of familiar possessions, most of which have special memories attached. In an odd kind of way, it feels as if I will disappear if my stuff does. Nevertheless, we combine and re-organize as best we can.

Learning to live together is harder than we had imagined. He is a minimalist, while I am a clutter bug. He's happy to eat out of a can, while I want a properly prepared meal. As the first few months go by, old baggage from our respective histories dumps crap for us to deal with. Even so, we persevere to make it work.

Aside from the adjustments of everyday living, the common ground we share enables us to find delight and laughter in leisure moments. Many are the meaningful discussions over meals and on trips out of town. In the fires of life's adversity, David's wisdom has been forged differently than mine, so we each bring diverse perspectives and experiences that we can learn from.

Finding a new meaning for my life is still proving to be elusive. I have sporadic periods of paid work mixed with bouts of being a dependent – not a comfortable position for either of us.

Time marches on; we celebrate my 60th birthday in March of 2010 with a party of dear friends and loved ones. How blessed I feel to be surrounded by so many who care about me.

In the past, whenever a new decade dawned, I usually challenged myself in some way to add to my personal or professional growth. At 40, I had taken singing lessons and writing classes. At 50, I'd enrolled in a stand-up comedy course and performed triumphantly at Yuk-Yuk's on Amateur Night. As I approach 60, no new ideas come to mind, which is why my next big challenge blindsides me one month before my 61st birthday.

There's that old saying that life happens when you're making other plans. Health-wise throughout my adult life, I had been plagued with constipation and hemorrhoids, but usually ignored the doctor's instructions to complete and submit those nasty occult blood tests.

It is February 2011. Suspicious rectal bleeding starts. I have ignored symptoms for several months. Finally, I visit my family doctor. She detects a mass that she thinks could be internal hemorrhoids. Just to be sure, she refers me to a consulting surgeon.

After a brief digital exam, the specialist, with his back to me, brusquely tells me that he is pretty sure I have a cancerous tumor and wants to confirm it with an emergency colonoscopy the next day. Shock triggers an instant numbness in both my mind and body. I can hardly breathe, never mind move. I barely hear his rapid-fire instructions as he leaves the room.

On my way out of the examination room, I stop by his desk to clarify the preparation procedure for the colonoscopy. One look at my face has him asking, "Are you alright?"

I want to scream, "Of course I'm not alright. You just told me you're sure I have cancer!" But politeness prevails, so I just nod and leave the building.

It was a mistake to drive myself to the appointment. As soon as I'm in my car, I start crying so hard I don't know how I'll see the road. Somehow, I make it home safely.

The next morning, David comes with me for the colonoscopy. The surgeon confirms his suspicions. I am diagnosed with anal cancer – a slow-growing tumor has revealed itself inside the canal near my rectum. At Stage 2, it is considered serious but not life- threatening.

Journal – March 2011

It's been five weeks since Cancer dragged me front and center and commanded me to dance. Those of you who have also been commanded to swing to this same music likely remember the terror and disbelief when you saw your name on that dance card.

The orchestra (a.k.a. Western Medicine) immediately struck up a whirling polka of more testing, consulting, and the resulting chat about what they soon planned to do to my body to eradicate the malignant cells. The most shocking news from the colonoscopy (in addition to the pictorial evidence of cancer) is that surgery is recommended – they would totally remove the rectal area and leave me with a colostomy bag for the rest of my life. While the doctor waits for biopsy results, he plans to refer me to the Cross Cancer Institute for their opinion about the alternatives of radiation and chemotherapy.

The week of waiting is a nightmare of feelings as I envision life after surgery. Every fiber of my being screams, "No, no, no!" David is quick to reassure me that he loves me for who I am; that a bag attached to me will not diminish his love for me nor affect my sexual attractiveness.

Family and friends are horrified when they hear my news. My name is added to countless prayer lists. While I feel grateful to be surrounded by so many people who care, I hate feeling so victimized.

A week later, we meet with the surgeon for the biopsy results. He delivers the best possible news – the biopsy revealed a type of cancer cell that responds well to radiation, so surgery will not be done after all. Our question is, "That's good news, right?" You can imagine my relief to have dodged the surgery bullet – not that I am out of the woods, but the future looks much brighter. My body wants to do the dance of joy down the hospital corridor.

At Cross Cancer, they do an MRI before I see the two oncologists who work as a team – first, the resident to give me the background, take my history and explain what she knows. After that, they conduct a physical exam, and the specialist weighs in with his thoughts and perspectives.

It seems as if they are both excited about having me as a new toy to do battle with cancer. When I suggest some wholistic alternatives to the oncologist, he is quick to dismiss my ideas as nonsense. Even though he can give no guarantees about his protocols, I am told that they have this cool, new radiation machine to use if I am willing to participate in their study to track the good, the bad, and the ugly bits of this current protocol.

Oh, and by the way, they will also inject a couple of deadly toxins (chemotherapy), just to make sure those nasty cells get what they deserve. The price of admission – innocent, healthy cells will also die. Plus, I'd be part of their research study for five years, with additional tests etc. as part of the process.

Hold it – stop the music! While the idea of cancer is scary to me, the thought of radiation and particularly chemo is terror personified. During the week between the colonoscopy and the referral to the Cross Cancer Institute, I had researched alternatives. I am not ready to turn myself over to their treatment, nor am I enamored of the arrogant attitude of the various specialists who poo-pooed my ideas for a different approach.

Since my twenties, I'd become fascinated with all types of alternative healing and had benefited from trying a few of them. And though I'd had a teenage stint as a junk food junkie, these past years I have become more conscious of putting healthier foods into my body – even to the point of testing vegan recipes.

I have also been drawn to explore the emotional aspect of cancer. One author defined it as fear of being oneself. I look up cancer in Louise Hay's book, Heal Your Body. It shows the reason for cancer as: "Deep hurt. Longstanding resentment. Deep secret or grief eating away at the self. Carrying hatreds. 'What's the use?'" I remember all my attempts to "keep a lid" on my true nature. My history clearly points to an issue in that arena.

I recall a defining event from childhood. I was four and had been instructed to keep a secret regarding a special Christmas gift for my dad. Forgetting it was a secret, I blurted it out the moment I saw him. Of course, Mom found out and went into a rage. Her punishment was swift and severe.

As an extremely sensitive child, a mere frown from an adult would send me scurrying to better behavior. So that level of correction quickly taught me that it was not safe to be my normal, boisterous, exuberant, self.

I remember at around age 5, I began the process of folding myself into an acceptable box. It took time and energy – years in fact, but I'd grown up with the adage "children should be seen and not heard", so I used that as my guide. I became quiet as a mouse – a good, obedient girl who was polite, helpful, and self-sacrificing.

Though I thought I would love school, I was terrified of our Grade One teacher. In those days, if you had to go to the bathroom, you printed your name on the chalk board before leaving the room. Only one person could go at a time. I hated that everyone in the class knew when I had to pee.

She was the only teacher in the school to have a leather strap in her desk. At the hint of any misbehavior, she didn't hesitate to use it. It's a mystery that I managed to escape that punishment, but I lived in fear of her ridicule and her wrath.

Most of the time, my efforts to subdue the real me worked; but every now and again, much to my dismay, the old Me would leak out. Like the time in Grade One when one of the boys threw up into the wastebasket. I was so upset for him that nervous laughter bubbled unbidden out of my mouth, earning me scorn from my classmates and a sharp reprimand from our teacher.

My grade two year was much better because I had a kind and gentle teacher who encouraged me and smiled a lot. What a relief!

We moved to the farm when I was eight, so I attended a country school for grade three. I quickly learned that my new classmates were much farther ahead with writing and reading. I struggled to catch up. It must have been a miserable time because at home, I started to wet the bed.

My mother didn't hesitate to show her disgust at someone my age soiling the bed sheets. I became even quieter, I rarely smiled, and I made the conscious decision to withhold affection from my parents. I stopped kissing them goodnight.

By grade four, I was unhappy enough to slide into a depressed state, though I doubt that depression was something they would have diagnosed in a child in those days. I developed bladder and kidney infections to the extent that my mother had to tell the teachers about my urgency to pee, so I could go when I needed to without them chastising me. When I look at birthday pictures of me during those years, I was rarely smiling, despite nice parties and gifts.

Life on the farm though provided the balm to help lift my spirits. Nature beckoned in spring with pussy willows, elusive garter snakes, and budding trees. I remember hot summer days where I'd pull myself atop of one of the haystacks and lie for hours just watching the clouds go by. There were trees to climb and books to read – books about daring acts of courage and independence – Lorna Doone, Pollyanna, Suzanna of the Mounties.

But it would not be until my twenties that I would begin to feel strong enough to allow the real me out of that self-imposed prison that I had built to keep me safe.

INVISIBLE©

Sitting there in the shadow of older and bigger voices,
she watched and listened.
Early life had taught her to hide her true self,
tone down her raucous laugh and boisterous nature. She did it to survive, to
feel safe, to be accepted.

In tiny parcels,
she sent her joyous loud parts to different places in her body,
with strict instructions to stay put and not bother her.

Every now and then, much to her horror,
an insane giggle would bubble its way to her throat
and burst forth unbidden.
Shame and guilt flooded her next as she struggled to regain control.

As she grew, it became harder to contain those unruly emotions.
Her body moaned with the pain of all that was stuffed inside –
joy and love, but mostly fear, anger, and sadness.
A part of her yearned for the freedom to be as she was meant,
but the bonds were tight – she had been invisible for so long.

At 24, without conscious knowing, she began to reclaim her Soul.
In safe havens of like-minded, her real Self began to emerge.
Most of the time, this battle for Being was messy and hard won.
Occasionally, a state of grace enabled her to accept this new self
freely and easily.

Oddly enough, it was tragedy and grief that caused the biggest shifts.
Pain proved a mighty tool for opening to Self.
Brick by brick, this prison of her making began to reshape itself.
Windows appeared, then doors with shafts of light streaming in.
She embraced the new-found light as she continued to open.

Surrender was the golden key that unlocked the doors of her heart.
"Thy will be done" became her mantra.
New muscles of forgiveness wrapped bitter tendons with love and caring.

This prison is now an ever-growing Temple,
where Self is cherished as a precious piece of the Cosmos
and Love is worshiped as the only way. "To thine own Self be true,"
she whispered.

Chapter 5

Maybe you are searching in the branches for
what only appears in the roots. **Rumi**

Bless the internet for its reams of information, not only about my type of cancer and the standard protocol of treatment, but for the vast array of alternative methods of healing that had substantial sources of scientific and anecdotal documentation.

The only thing I know for sure is that I don't want to make any decisions about treatment that are based on fear. I am starting to suspect that it isn't the cancer itself, but the fear of cancer and the fear of having cancer, and the fear of dying a horrible death because of cancer that creates panic and depression and stops most people from taking charge of their healing.

In response to my diagnosis, my friend, Gladys sends me a book title that she believes is must-read. The book, Knock-Out, by Suzanne Somers is an eye opener. It is filled with information from traditional oncologists who had turned from Western therapies – surgery, chemo and radiation, and found less invasive methods to help the body heal.

I find comfort in the idea that each person needs to decide about the treatment that he/she believes will support the healing process. If you believe that chemo and radiation is what will work for you, then that's what you pick. It's your choice.

I, however, can't see the sense in destroying my immune system in order to eradicate the cancer cells. I had learned over the years that our bodies are miraculous in their ability to grow and heal, particularly when given the best chance to do so.

Since I also hold some deep-seated beliefs about the mind-body-spirit connection, I want to identify ways to treat my whole being, not just the malignant cells that are having a party at my expense. I believe I have an intense time of soul-searching and visualization ahead to determine what course of action feels right for me.

At this point in my story, it might be helpful for you to understand a little about my journey as a spiritual quester. From the time I was introduced to God as a small child while saying prayers at bedtime, I wanted to know more. My earliest recollection of learning about God, Jesus, and the Bible was at about the age of 8. Mom decided we needed some religious teaching. Even though she wouldn't go to church with us, nor would my father, a staunch Agnostic, we were sent up the hill to Sunday School at the Baptist Church – the closest one to our farm.

The congregation was kind to us, and we enjoyed participating in summer picnics and winter tobogganing outings. When they discovered my brother's sweet soprano voice, he sang in the choir – even doing a solo at Christmas. I, in turn, got my first applause in church when I memorized and recited a poem one Sunday.

I remember struggling to understand the difference between God and Jesus. Who exactly was I supposed to pray to, and if I made the wrong choice, would my prayers still be answered? As for reading the Bible, I wanted to be a diligent student, so I started at page one of Genesis.

I confess that all that begetting eventually got to me; my goal of reading the Bible from cover to cover was soon replaced by guilt at not doing what was supposed to be very good for me.

Likely my parents were dismayed by the sanctimonious preaching of their nine-year-old as I struggled to sort out what was a sin and what was not. Intentions and behaviors seemed to be at odds with the teachings!

Our Baptist adventure didn't last that long, as Mom was an Anglican by upbringing and confirmation.

During junior high, my girlfriend, Holly, whose family was also Anglican, joined me in the trek to Edmonton for weekly confirmation classes. There, as we memorized "The Creed", we were taught that we were the most miserable sinners, whose only salvation was through the church. I was uneasy about learning text that I didn't believe. But I was in no position to rebel.

Rev. Ledbetter was a kind and patient man, who helped us with the all-important verbiage, which we would have to recite, letter-perfect, to be confirmed.

Shallow though it may seem, the best part of getting confirmed was the lovely dress my mother bought me and the delicate string of pearls that we picked out together as my gift. Confirmation Day brought warm summer sun. We had the photo opp. on the farm with the family all spruced up and gathered round.

At church, no hitches or glitches marred the dignity of the occasion, and all of us received our certificates. Anglicans use real wine for communion, so that was likely my first taste of spirits – for spiritual purposes only!

For years after, though I didn't attend church regularly, when I did go, I found that I was offended at having to recite that I was a miserable sinner. I didn't believe that I was that much of a sinner – after all, how much sinning could a 14-year-old do who was too afraid to follow anything other than the code, "Let your conscience be your guide"? Of course, those doubts about the teachings triggered some guilt.

Rather than finding comfort and solace in religious teachings, I had a rather uneasy relationship with God. It seemed logical to me that he would be my friend, as would his son, but too many Bible stories pointed to his wrath and vengeful nature. Would I go straight to hell if I believed what made sense to me, even if it was at odds with what I'd been taught?

There was really no one I could ask about my doubts and my musings. Religion and politics were two taboo topics in our household – oh, and sex – that subject was never even whispered, never mind talked about!

I just kept quiet as I played the role of dutiful churchgoer. Fortunately, my discomfort didn't arise too often, as we were not a family of diligent attendees. Sundays in the summer were often spent on the golf course. Church was reserved for

Easter and Christmas, and the occasional wedding or funeral.

In grade 9, I borrowed a book from the library on Buddhist philosophy. It was a tough, yet intriguing read – my first glimpse into a life that was vastly different from the one I lived. Although I lost interest before finishing it, the book left its mark. The other book that filled me with wonderment in those days was Kahlil Gibran's "The Prophet". His poetry stirred longings in my adolescent soul, even though I didn't understand it all.

Eventually I made a pact with God. He would listen to my prayers – maybe even grant a few requests - and keep me safe from harm. I, in turn, would do what I was told, get good marks in school, be kind and serve others, and above all, not cause trouble.

That pact was broken the day my mother died suddenly of a cerebral hemorrhage. After a mysterious illness at home, she had been diagnosed with leukemia just days earlier. Before I could say goodbye, she was gone. I was 17.

Betrayal was the word that struck me as I began to feel the depth of that loss. I'd spent years trying to be "Miss Goodie Two Shoes". I'd been a dutiful daughter – sacrificing, respectful, giving – the behavior that was supposed to grant me safe passage through life. God was in charge of that – right? If he was so powerful, then why would he take my mother away? How could he just let my family shatter? If you couldn't trust God, then who could you trust?

Those thoughts warred with my worry and feelings of guilt that despite all attempts, I had somehow not measured up – in the eyes of God, I wasn't quite worthy enough to be kept safe.

As I had once inwardly shut out my parents, I then turned away from God. If following all those rules wouldn't keep me safe, then I would follow my own rules – tackle the world on my own terms. I was angry enough that had I known the F-word – I might have stuck my middle finger up to the heavens and shouted, "Fuck You!"

There was a fascinating kind of freedom in that self-determination. It grew into a fierce independence. Despite my naiveté and lack of worldly experience, I vowed to succeed. Though I accepted and appreciated all the help I got from family, friends, and strangers along the way, I still felt alone and isolated in my journey through life – caught somehow in that neutral zone between who I had been and who I was to become.

At 23, my world was rattled once again when I was fired from a dicta-typing/reception job with an insurance company. I had been working toward a position as a full-fledged secretary – the only career I felt was open to me at the time. I was reasonably competent but lacked the sitability the job required. Frustrated, I planned to turn in my notice. I was mad when they fired me before I got the chance to quit.

Once my tears dried, I scoured the want ads, determined that if there was no such thing as job security, I would make my own. One small ad for a Holiday Girl appealed to me. As an independent saleswoman for Holiday Magic Cosmetics, I would sell beauty products to women, door-to-door.

Part of the training was an introduction to the book, *Think & Grow Rich*, by Napoleon Hill. I was fascinated by his ideas and the resulting stories of success. Weekly sales meetings pumped us up to use our energy to succeed. Some months later, the company offered a personal growth program called, *Mind Dynamics*.

Attending that workshop opened the door to an enlightenment and sense of personal power I had not known existed. In four long days and five subsequent evenings, I learned that I was a person in my own right; that I could choose my own destiny and was, in fact, responsible for it.

Harnessing the power of the subconscious mind was a major key to locking in dreams and goals. Active meditation was the tool we used for transforming imagination into reality. Through guided visualizations and internal experiences, I began the healing process of forgiving my parents, of reconciling the loss of my family, of discovering who I really was. Small victories emerged as I practiced the tools. My day-to-day life ran more smoothly. Hope shone as a daily ray of bright sunshine.

Anytime we journey into Self, there can be the fear of discovering and confirming the demons, the shadow side of ourselves that we fear might lurk behind closed doors. During the training, that opportunity to explore presented itself. Scared though I was, I opened the door, certain that I could deal with every bit of the bad in me.

Much to my surprise and delight, there were no demons – only Me – pure and delightful. Any yucky stuff was dealt with and cast off, like old clothes. This re-birth felt much as I imagine butterflies feel after struggling to escape the confines of their cocoons. I had new wings, and I was ready to soar.

However, I was pretty selective about whom I chose to share this remarkable adventure with. (It was 1974 after all.) I did apply some heavy pressure to Wayne, my first husband – we married in 1968 – just a year after my mother died.

Since the course had worked so well for me, then surely it would pull him out of his depression and inability to find himself. It could even save our marriage. I wanted Wayne to get the same things I had – and I wanted to be able to share this growth path with him. Much to my dismay, he attended three-quarters of the training and quit at a crucial point. He remained in his misery, his key to freedom out of reach.

Torn between my need to grow and my duty to him and our marriage, I set aside the teachings for a time. When I was desperate for help with some issue, I would meditate in private and then carry on with life.

Three years later, with all attempts at rescuing our relationship having failed, I moved in with an aunt and uncle to re-group and decide on my next course of action. It didn't take long for me to re-enter the personal growth arena. I took the basic course again, and then signed up for the more advanced *Interpersonal Experience* – six full days of intensive self- exploration. I also began to journal, calling my entries: *Learning to Love Susan.*

My personal growth journey continued throughout the years as I took courses, read the latest books, and practiced whatever I thought would help me grow and improve. A couple of mystical experiences along the way had me re-examining my connection to God.

During one women's retreat on the theme of Joy, our facilitator guided us through a deep meditation where I soared to the heavens and saw the face of God. I had trouble believing what I had seen and voiced that to our leader. She replied, "Who are you to deny seeing God?"

The next morning as I walked the shores of the lake by our facility, I was struck by the peace of the scene before me – a slight mist rising from the glassy surface of the water, loons swimming by gracefully. A voice whispered, "This is Joy – whether you choose to participate or not is up to you."

That experience had me doubling my efforts to improve myself. While I hoped there was a place for me, I felt very separate and alone. I believed that if I could just grow enough, get good enough, then I'd be worthy of being brought into the fold and would become part of God.

My near-death experience in 2007 blew that theory right out the window. Contrary to my former beliefs, I felt and experienced with
all the certainty of my being that I had always and would always be a treasured part of God – not because I'd done anything to deserve it, but because it was my birthright for Being. I was a part of Spirit who was as amazing and essential as anyone else was. The separation I'd been feeling was self-induced and only existed in my mind.

Rather than needing to improve, my experience revealed that I was perfect in every way – magnificent, in fact. Nor did Death scare me, because I knew that only my body would be cast off at the end of my life – my Spirit would live on eternally.

While I did not fear death, the cancer treatment they were offering did terrify me. I searched for another way.

Chapter 6

We must accept finite disappointment, but never lose infinite hope.   Martin Luther King, Jr.

My prospective oncologists frown at the idea of alternative therapy, claiming they know nothing about it; in fact, they try to talk me out of it. But after a day at Cross Cancer where I am steeped in an atmosphere of fear, I just can't face being part of their invasive protocol.

I am horrified and distraught at the thought of daily radiation to a very vulnerable part of my anatomy, combined with the reality of ingesting deadly toxins. What is even harder to contemplate is being surrounded by other "victims" of cancer –who won't likely be feeling either happy or optimistic.

With my sensitive, empathic nature, I know that level of emotional bombardment will not be helpful at all. I bawl all the way home and scream at God and the Universe, "I'm not like them, I don't want to be like them!"

When I share the details of my day, David has tears in his eyes. "I don't want to lose you," he says. We talk through the options. His rational, logical mind helps me lay the foundation to sift through the vast array of information. I need to decide. "What do you think I should do?" I ask David. His opinion is to do it all – the radiation and chemo, plus whatever alternative treatments made the most sense.

With my intention to come to a peace about whatever I decide, I tuck in for the night. Sleep is replaced with me mentally and emotionally traveling down each path that we had discussed earlier in the evening. It's odd, but I feel divinely guided because of a sense of certainty that regardless of the path I choose, it isn't possible to make a "wrong" decision.

For most of my life it seems that my path has been one of survival. I'd struggled and clawed my way through a variety of circumstances until I achieved some success. More success than my comfort zone allowed had me starting over with something else.

Much like those steep old playground slides with the metal steps, I'd climb and climb, then pause at the top where I could see for miles. It was exhilarating and scary at the same time. Then I'd take that swift ride to the bottom and start the climb over again.

But at some point (I likely earned three PhDs in the school of survival) the satisfaction from the scratching and clawing was gone. I begin to wonder about the notion of what I have come to call **thrival**. What if my journey involves growth through ongoing bliss and joy? Abundance instead of lack; excitement instead of fear is one thing I want to strive for.

The radiation and chemo route seems to be one of survival laced with large doses of fear. Once I enter that arena, I will be consumed by everything to do with my cancer. In my dreamtime, I know that I could do it, that my body will survive it. But the price will be high emotionally, and if the treatments compromise certain healthy cells such as proper bowel and bladder function, my quality of life will change dramatically.

When I envision the alternative health route, there is no less effort to heal, but I believe the experience will be vastly different, both emotionally and physically. The quest I had begun some four years earlier to create and experience a life of ecstasy will continue. Healing my cancer is part of that journey.

I wake the next morning with a profound peace about my decision to turn away from modern medicine's dubious remedy and support my healing in a more natural and less invasive way. When asked about my level of conviction in that decision, I respond with an immediate, "98%". I can hear David's gulp of fear as he states that he will support me in this decision, no matter what. Bless his heart!

Voice mail is a wonderful tool when you don't want pushback about decisions. That morning, I phone the respective oncology offices about my decision and leave my message. I then continue my research about alternative therapies.

I read about intravenous Vitamin C, ozone therapy, the alkaline diet, wheat grass juice and liver cleanses. Some therapies involve traveling thousands of miles, but many can be done right at home.

My Journal - June 2011

I explore emotional, mental, spiritual, and physical protocols. Some of it I can do myself. Other therapies will require practitioners' support. I'm confused about what to choose. How will I know what will work, and when will I know that it's working? Should I try just one thing at a time and assess results, or try multiple things at once? I feel like a live lab rat caught in a maze with no discernible way out.

Emotionally I start to ponder the idea that I created MY cancer. Do I need to take full ownership and full responsibility for this condition in my body? I can feel my resistance to this because it feels as if, in taking full responsibility for its creation, I will also need to take the blame for it. Who would do this horrific thing to themselves and their loved ones?

On a spiritual level, I toy briefly with the idea that my eternal Self had laid the foundation for the creation of cancer – all to further my growth on the physical plane. Hmmm – I don't know where to go with that thought.

As a human in my daily physical realm, I don't believe I knowingly, deliberately decided that cancer would be part of my life. Certainly, I fear cancer, as I think most people do – largely because of the media attention this disease attracts and the horrors that are experienced from current treatments.

However, whether through mental and emotional choices and circumstances, a Soul pact, or previous dietary and exercise habits, the fact remains that inside my body there is now a perfect environment for rogue cells to adopt the cancer persona.

*I've been beating myself up about having cancer – swinging from victimhood – why did this happen to me? – to – what's wrong with me that I would have created this? Then I worry about not doing enough to heal, feeling that I need to prove to myself and others that I can heal **my** way rather than the conventional way - that death won't be the ultimate victor.*

The path seems endless at times as I stumble along, unsure about my decisions. I am too afraid to not try all the various protocols – what if the one I turn away from is the "right" one? So much for not making decisions based on fear. When cancer takes hold, fear is the real enemy.

In my best moments, clarity comes that this cancer journey is perfect in all its imperfections. I delight in the taste sensations of fresh, living vegetables and fruits and bask in the warmth of David's love. But all that fails to provide any lasting solace.

Fears of the unknown pile up as does my impatience to be done with the journey and move on. I also feel simmering anger at having created cancer in the first place. Compelled to manage by myself as I've always done, I don't really trust what I'm doing, plus I know so little about most of the experimental methods. David has done tons of research and helps as much as I will allow. My determination to call my own shots is not born from knowing exactly what to do and how to do it.

Uncertainty about my future sharpens my daily senses. Both a heightened awareness and more bursts of gratitude fill the times in my day when I am not focused on my work or on my healing.

What surprises me is the fear I hear in the doctors' voices. They are as scared of my path of healing as I am of their treatment. They are also deathly afraid of cancer, these warriors in white coats. Truth be told, they know they lose more battles than they win, despite increasingly high-tech equipment and the promises of the drug companies. For them, regardless of cost, death is the enemy to fight.

I guess I've stared death in the face too many times to be that afraid of it. There are worse things than being dead. Worse is turning over the control of my body to a group of complete strangers who are arrogant enough to think they know what is best for me. They might have "a" way to treat this, but I doubt they have "the" way.

I hear about and then read Brandon Bey's books that describe how she had healed herself when she had a large tumor. She offers hope and a methodology that worked for her. I feel hopeful for the same healing. In our most spiritually connected moments, David and I channel healing energy into my body. It feels great, but I have no way of knowing if it is working.

The research on high doses of Intravenous Vitamin C is convincing. A Canadian scientist had proven that a minimum of 45 grams of C given intravenously works to kill cancer cells. I find a clinic and start the therapy. I also start a new food protocol based on the results of a live blood cell analysis.

Chapter 7

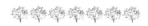

Always seek out the seeds of triumph in every adversity.   **Og Mandino**

My Journal

July 2011

Cracks in David's and my relationship emerge along with the mounting costs of alternative treatments. Intravenous Vitamin C in large doses costs over $300/week. I am not carrying my financial weight in our partnership – he does not want me to consider the cost and the resulting toll, but I sense his worry and can't help but worry, too. I feel trapped, yet ready to leave if David's too unhappy.

We both care deeply for one another, but our different ways of being and doing combined with my scary health situation cause us both anguish.

July 28, 2011

I have my third live blood cell analysis – good results in that my candida has dropped again - from level 4 to a 2 – of course 1 is the lowest rating. My body responds positively to the new food protocol not only with weight loss but an increasing sense of vitality.

A week or so after the live cell test, I continue working with my buddy Pam, a nurse and alternative healer who is skilled at several different emotional healing protocols. She helps me integrate and release any current distress around various challenges.

We muscle test the IV C and ozone therapy for my August treatments. How blessed I am to have found her to contribute to my healing path. Almost every day in some way or another I use the Sensory Evolution Technique (SET) that I learned in a workshop to balance myself. Of course, the results are always stronger when I have Pam's help with it.

My third urine sample goes off to the Philippines for analysis. So much has happened spiritually since the good results from the last one that I feel confident that the markers will have dropped again significantly.

August 12, 2011

Full moon – I wake up knowing that it's been too long since I've written about my journey and my feelings. Such progress I've made! I worked with Pam about a week ago. She used a couple of new techniques from

SET to help with my healing. One was a centering spot in the belly, just below the diaphragm. I was wound up tighter than a top, with a gassy feeling in my chest. I also found it hard to take a deep breath. After several rounds of setting and re-setting my points, I began to feel much better.

The finish line then is the third urine test which I completed on Saturday plus, the upcoming MRI on September 8. It will be seven months less one day since my original diagnosis. I'm ready to move on now to my new life, with a new career and a deeper relationship with David.

I'm not the same person I was a year ago. I've shed 40 lbs. and look healthier and younger than I have for years. I've discovered the joys of raw vegetables and treat my body more like the temple that it is.

In the mirror, I marvel at the woman I see – slim, sexy, youthful – who would guess my 61 years?! My self-care has increased 10-fold as I meditate and get more exercise. I'm even becoming more disciplined in my approach to the tasks at hand, whether work-related, house-related or focused on my own care.

It's funny that along the way I've turned so inward, relinquishing some of my need to rescue others – surrendering them to their own paths and beginning to trust that they'll sort it out themselves or get help from another source if I can't do it (or don't choose to).

Now it feels as if a new leg of my journey begins. I have left my body's old house with all its burdens and woes and wiped the proverbial slate clean; except I retain the wisdom I've gathered along the way. Hopefully I can leave the fears, too. This new path is one of potential joy and discovery.

September 6, 2011

It's been an unsettling time as the date of my MRI approaches. My urine test results show a disappointing rise in markers instead of a decrease. Our road trip last week to see my family in Calgary and in Brooks hit me harder emotionally than I would have guessed.

It was the first time my birth family had seen me since my diagnosis. I saw and sensed both deep love and fear for me in my dad's and my brother's eyes. In some ways it's as if they are seeing me for the first time in a long while – as the person I am today– a daughter, a sister who is struggling with the threat of death.

Bless them. They may have been fearful of the healing path I have chosen, but they respect my decision and continue to give me all their support.

I feel threatened by my looming MRI. I haven't felt good all week – an internal tiredness zaps my spark. I'm unsure of my next step if the results are worse instead of better. Feeling as I have this past week, I doubt my strength to continue the fight. I'm weepy and feeling vulnerable. Everything seems such an effort. I'm struggling to do my part. I'm afraid it's more than just feeling punk from travel and all the emotions stirred up when with my family.

David and I start getting excited about a new business venture. We're also more connected than we've been in several months. I know now as I've sensed but never really felt before that he will do anything for me – give me the moon and the stars, because of his love for me. There's a part of my old unworthiness that is afraid I'll reject his incredible gift by doing something insane like dying instead of us growing very old together.

But thoughts of a bright future also beg for attention. I don't think I'm ready to cash in my chips. An old memory of a workshop on the meaning of life bubbles to the surface. I had attended when I was 27. In one exercise, we were to imagine ourselves dead, hovering over our own funerals. Who was there and what were they saying?

I remember bursting into tears later as I shared with the group. The thought of leaving all that I cherished – family, sunsets, green grass, the wonders of Mother Earth was unbearable. I realize that I'm not ready to leave it now, either.

I focus on what I want for my new future:

I want to be vibrating with health and energy, with all cancer cells gone and my lesion healed – to be at peace with my body, trusting it to support me as I support it.

I want to leave my mark on planet Earth in a more visible and significant way – a way that helps others out of the depths of their fears and into the light of their own magnificence.

I want to finish my memoirs. I want to complete the fantasy novel I started for my future grandchildren.

I want to travel to more parts of the world – experiencing the wonder of other people and places.

I want to financially support causes and people I believe in. I want to write a play – a musical – and have it produced.

Why do I want all of this? Because I want the feeling of satisfaction that I can do all of it – that is thriving – missing nothing that is important to me in life.

I also want to right the balance in my life – to move spiritually, emotionally, and physically from the constant struggles I have grown up with into a new life filled with joy and ecstasy.

My cancer has been one born of old hurts, fears, and unforgiveness that fester and eat away at me. No more, no more. Here and now, I want to release it all, burn the pages of all past sins of mine and all others, relinquishing the need to harbor old resentments and sadness.

Why, I ask again, do I want all I describe? Because I'm worthy. Because I choose to step into the next best version of me, someone who is having the greatest adventure possible.

September 13, 2011

I had my MRI yesterday and brought the films home of both this one and the one from February. Of course, we have no what we were looking at when we go over all the images, so can only guess at the results.

I woke up this morning feeling different. The weight of the MRI is gone, and I feel that no matter the results, I'm moving forward with peace and joy. I don't plan to give my cancer any more weight in my life than I give to the rest of what's important to me.

I want to trust that my body knows how to heal itself, so as I provide it with the tools to do so, it will do just that. In the meantime, I will carry on with the rest of what's important to me – new work that I love and the building of my relationship with my partner.

I'm taking a break from IV C and ozone this week and will work with Pam instead. Then we'll test dosages and frequencies for those two, so I know where I'm at. I'm thinking some wheat grass enemas might be appropriate, though I have no clue how to do them.

On my journey to full health, I'm committed to living my life without that specter of fear about the cancer cells in my body. How blessed I am that David initiates healing meditations and whatever else he can to support my health and happiness.

Chapter 8

*Your pain is the breaking of the shell that encloses
your understanding.*
Khalil Gibran, *The Prophet*

On September 20, the news from the MRI is devastating. The tumor has grown in the last seven months, not shrunk as I had hoped. I don't know how to carry on. Has it all been a waste? Have I made the biggest mistake of my life by not turning myself over to the radiation and chemo doctors?

I have been so confident in my path, and my body responded well for at least five months. But I have not felt as good the past while – tired with some bothersome sensations in my tailbone area. All I've done to heal has not seemed to make the slightest difference to the tumor.

A part of me wants to just give up. I am scared to try anything else – what was supposed to happen with vitamin C intravenous has not worked. Nor has the ozone therapy or alkaline diet.

It's been a long seven months, fraught with struggles to change and stick to healing protocols. I find myself tired of the fight – how do people keep on for years and years?

Four years ago, I could have just slipped away, peacefully bled to death, and just left this world in a gentle and undisturbed way. Did I come back only to die a cruel and miserable death from this cancer that brings tremendous pain and heartache to me and all those I know and love?

How could I be on the brink of having the wonderful life I've always dreamed of, only to have it snatched away for no reason I can possibly understand? I've done the work, come to peace with so many things. I'm a good person – I don't deserve this crap. It's too cruel a joke to play even on someone's worst enemy. Fuck off cancer and just leave me alone!

I don't know how much more I can give to this. It makes no sense to me – I can't see my way out and I am scared of burdening my lover and the rest of my family with caring for a weak and pathetic creature. I don't know who or what to trust – I don't seem to be able to trust myself to make the right decisions – how could a decision that felt so right in March turn out so wrong?

I can't bear to give my family and friends yet more bad news. David has been my rock through all this – what would I have done without him? Yet it seems so unfair to put him through all this anguish. I'm afraid I'll become a dependent, not his equal. He deserves a fully functioning partner. What if I can't be that?

If I agree to radiation, it will supposedly kill the cancer cells, so the tumor won't grow. I need to trust that the radiation won't do irreparable damage to the muscles and tissues in the bladder, vagina, and anal canal. I've heard some horror stories, and I certainly don't want to be one of them. Perhaps if I do IV C along with the treatments, that will mitigate some damage.

But if I continue to work with different alternative treatments, I need support from a doctor with the ability to test what is working and provide ongoing support. There's been so much uncertainty because each person I have consulted has pieces of the puzzle that supposedly fit, but no one seems to know where all the pieces are to complete the healing picture. I just don't know where to turn or what to do next.

My Journal October 18, 2011

It's been a whirlwind of thoughts and activity since my last entry. I quit my old naturopathic clinic after I discovered that there had been a huge mistake in the dosage calculation for my IV C. I was getting too low a dose to kill cancer cells.

I demanded and got a refund and then found a new clinic, the Optimum Wellness Center that has a much more professional approach to working with patients – especially cancer patients. Dr. DeNault, the Naturopath has the pharmaceutical background to know how to combine their alternative therapy with radiation and chemo. It's a huge relief to turn the management of my healing protocol over to this skilled practitioner.

My second trip to the Cross is very different. I meet a new oncologist. Young and respectful, Dr. Usmani listens to me with great care and concern. I get the kid-glove treatment – likely he has read about my defiance in the report of my first visit! Even though he is filling in for the first oncologist I saw, he gives me the option of keeping him as my doctor. I say yes.

While I will continue the Vitamin C treatments, I will turn myself over to the radiation and chemo doctors. Despite my misgivings, I believe I can survive the treatment.

Treatments at the Cross Cancer start on Halloween – how odd is that! I've certainly looked at both as a person's worst nightmare – especially my worst nightmare. I will get all the tricks – with nary a treat in sight - dammit.

However, when the doctor gives me the stats for my type of cancer using radiation - a 72% cure rate with no reoccurrence, I am very encouraged. They have good results with the new machine that will be used – more targeted and lower dosages of radiation needed with fewer side effects. I can now enter Cross with much more peace than my first visit last February. I feel my attitude shift from one of distrust to one of cautious trust – that the healers who will work with me are the best ones for my situation.

On the spiritual front, I keep getting the message that me waging a "war" on my tumor is not the right approach. All those wonky cells are as bereft of love as I have been. In my visualizations, I will shine light and love on all of them, so that the ones that can transform into healthy ones will do so, the ones too damaged, will slough off.

Spoon Bending

Thoughts about personal power and control surface as I face this next step. Initially, it seems as if I will lose all control if I turn my body over to Cross and let them do their worst. I am so afraid to do the radiation/chemo, yet equally scared not to. And because I no longer believe I know enough about what else might work, I don't feel competent to manage or to heal through alternatives – a definite control issue!

I believe, at the core of it all is my sense of personal power. When I'm feeling most powerful, I can choose to consciously turn control over to those whom I pick to be of service.

This sense of personal power has been a long time in coming. In the 1970s when I taught personal growth seminars, one of the ways we helped people experience the height of their personal power was to show them how to bend spoons using the power of their minds. It's such a cool thing to do, even though it often freaks people out. What can come from that success is an eagerness to test other boundaries. "Because I can do that, what else can I do?" (Quantum Physics has since proved that spoon bending is not just a party trick!)

Not long after I got the cancer diagnosis, I remembered my old spoon- bending days. Because I had succeeded at that seemingly impossible task in my past, I believed that I could turn my attention to the cancer and do the same thing.

Horror of horrors, when I tried and failed to bend my spoon, I lost my confidence in my own power. It seeded the fear that the cancer was bigger than me – that it had more power than I did.

On September 24, a former student of mine from my old Mind Dynamics/spoon bending days, Lezlie Molyneux, died suddenly from a brain tumor. Since that first class, Lezlie and I had become dear friends and shared many spiritual thoughts and life adventures over the years. Four years younger than I, she had faced dark times with courage and determination – winning when many thought the odds were impossible.

We had just had dinner with Ron and Lezlie in July. So, it was a huge shock to hear that she was gone. But somehow, despite my sadness for her family and my own sadness, I felt that she had chosen to go when she did so she could assist us better from the higher realms. Her celebration of life service was a moving tribute to the woman she was. A couple of her quotes stuck in my mind – "I have no time for fear" was one of them.

The other one was – "I have learned that I have no control over anything other than my capacity to love and ability to give it."

At her service, we were encouraged to take a rock from the pile that had been gathered from the Vancouver Island beach where Lezlie loved to roam. I put it in my purse as my talisman.

About a week after the funeral, Lezlie visits me in my dreams. She tells me emphatically to just go bend that spoon! I feel her love, her strength, and her confidence in me. I awake from the dream, pad downstairs, and find a big serving spoon in the drawer. I focus on it, stroke it, and seconds later feel it bend like soft taffy. My power is back! I leave it on the kitchen counter as evidence and go back to bed.

When he sees the bent spoon on the counter the next morning, David asks, "What do you think would happen if you bent a spoon every day for the next month?" I stock up on spoons and forks from the Dollar Store, determined to strengthen my confidence in my power. I also decide to flood my tumor with love and light whenever it came to mind.

Still scared, I feel I can move ahead despite that fear.

Chapter 9

It is during our darkest moments that we must focus to see the light. **Aristotle Onassis**

My Journal

November 6, 2011

The first week of chemo and radiation is done. It has been a horrible week – adjusting to the idea, never mind the reality of treatments every day in addition to coping with daily living. David doesn't handle it well – too much pressure on all sides- managing two businesses without any help, struggling with the financial strain, and dealing with his own feelings. He needs someone to talk to who is distanced from our situation.

My heart weeps to see him suffering so. It will be a bleak future indeed if we can't find ourselves and each other at the end of this whole trauma.

But in the meantime, my job is to heal. I'm using SET to deal with some nausea. I'm very tired and need to combine good rest with activity and exercise. It looks as if I can start the Vitamin C on Wednesday – I'm hoping that will provide a much-needed boost.

My side effects so far are mild – some gum tenderness, mild nausea, soreness, and redness in the skin around the radiation site. My lower abdomen is tender. I'll have to re-read which effects come from the chemo and which from the radiation.

My weight is stable – a good sign, but I need to make sure I'm eating enough, even though I'm not hungry. On the business front, despite extreme tiredness, I marshal every ounce of energy I have for the business trade show we book to demonstrate our products.

What a relief that our small booth generates success beyond our expectations – we book at least a dozen solid appointments. The goal is to generate some cash flow and some raving fans, with referral possibilities. I'll do what I can, but my energy is so unpredictable; I'm not sure I'm up for handling the scheduled appointments. For now, I may only be able to cheer and support from the sidelines.

*If we can have some wins with these calls, there will be some
hope for the future.*

November 25, 2011

*I've come through my treatment schedule far enough to have
my hair falling out at a rapid rate. Struggling with the
horror of losing my hair, I don't want to be constantly
finding clumps in the sink. Why let my hair die its own slow
death? So, contrary to my usual habit of just postponing the
inevitable, I take action.*

*Twenty minutes in the wig salon at Cross - my hair is all
gone – down to velvety fuzz, one-eighth of an inch long. The
young woman with the razor declares that I have no funny
bumps or odd-looking lumps on my skull and in fact my head
looks quite cute.*

*I don't know how I feel – a bit numb and detached. Have I joined
the ranks of cancer victims or cancer survivors? Is the label
appropriate at all? How quick we are to judge people and
situations based on what we observe or believe to be true.*

*What is true is that while wearing my wig, I can pretend for a
little while that I am normal – no funny stares from strangers
wondering what has been happening to me. Bless my
partner's heart for thinking and commenting that I'm
beautiful – that's not what I see when I look in the mirror. I
see the lines of fatigue, the lack of color in my cheeks, and a
strange, bald head.*

December 18, 2011

*This was supposed to be our day of Christmas celebrating with
our kids – turkey and all the trimmings, plus presents exchanged.
A trip on December 7 to Emergency at the Misericordia and then
a transfer to Cross changes all that.*

*Since December 8, I've been in a bed at the Cross. The fever
I'd been warned about happens, along with severe weakness
signals of a big infection brewing – a nasty yet known side*

effect. With no immune system left to fight, I am at risk of dying – not from cancer, but from the treatments.

Blood tests show a seriously low count on most fronts. The groin burns from the radiation are raw and sore. The doctor is glad we'd reserved a bed at the Cross two weeks before, just in case. How grateful I am for their special care.
They postpone radiation treatments until my blood counts rise to an acceptable level. My pain medication – morphine in high doses – causes delusion. Ever the storyteller, even I can hear me telling downright lies! They switch me to an engineered brand with fewer side effects but much more potency.

While I have no pain, it's been a nightmare of crisis as side effects from the morphine stopped up my poor bowels. It took two enemas and some agonizing time in the bathroom to get me unplugged. I want to just scream, but I can't do that to my roommate. That unplugging triggers diarrhea, which is still a challenge.

They send the burn team down to assess me. Their help and diligent care of my radiation burns provides almost full healing, plus a lot more comfort when sitting. As I write this, I'm sitting in a proper chair, with my feet on a low footstool, after days of being flat on my back. My poor tailbone isn't protesting much at all!

I have lots of visitors – nicely spaced so I can rest. Ta-ee-a, my friend and a professional caregiver sees to my comfort on her frequent visits. My son, Trevor drops by every few days on his way home from work. I'm so grateful for his time. We talk about mundane things, a relief from all my trials and tribulations. I ask him to do some Christmas shopping for me.

My one trip home on a day pass so I could participate in tree decorating and gather some things I need at the hospital is a good test to see what I am capable of and whether I will be able to manage at home.

Well, I can't. There are too many stairs to cope with. I just don't have the strength to do the self-care, be concerned about meals, plus heal through lots of resting. It's hard enough just to eat the meals they put before me at the hospital.

So I decide to save my passes for the 2-3 days of Christmas celebration. Hopefully, with all the sleeping I've been doing, I'll have more energy, despite the resumption of radiation treatments. It's hard to know what other side effects will pop up and what will be needed to deal with them. I'm just thankful to have the nursing staff to work their miracles.

Out of all of this, despite the pain and trauma resulting from treatment, I have this abiding, unshakable faith that this cure I've been promised has already happened. Even through the last of the radiation treatments, I can start to re-claim my body and steer it back to more perfect health.

More and more I'm trusting that the Universe will deliver what I need, when I need it, and in the quantity that's most beneficial for my body. It's that surrendering to the moment and allowing what needs to happen next.

Christmas 2011

December 23 marks my last radiation treatment – I prepare to go home for a small celebration. Joy, my cherished friend from Calgary arrives to spend Christmas with us. It's a lovely feast, but one I feel too tired to enjoy much. I realize I can't cope at home, so I head back to the hospital for my last days until discharge.

My brothers, Stew and Greg drive from Calgary for a visit. How glad I am to see them! If they are shocked at how I look, they don't show it. Greg shows me the game "Angry Birds" on his I-pad. I laugh and laugh at how funny it is. Their visit is much too short.

The next day I'm sent home. They've delivered their worst and done their best to eradicate my cancer. Now it's up to me. After being surrounded by help and support at the hospital, I feel strangely bereft and alone at home. It's like having my anchor cut and being all adrift.

The two flights of stairs are a huge challenge. I climb those 14 stairs as if I'm 103, with two rests partway up. Neither can I sit for very long, even in my comfy recliner. My computer, with the hundreds of e-mails awaiting reply collects more dust.

Along with healing, my goal is to wean myself off the high doses of my pain drugs. I worry about the telltale shaking in my body just before my next dose is due combined with the blissful release that kicks in when the pill takes effect. I am afraid of becoming addicted, but I can't tell if the lousy way I am feeling is because of the aftermath of radiation and chemo or the side effects from the dilaudid.

When I download from the internet the sheet of side effects and withdrawal symptoms of the drug, I am shocked at how many of them I have been experiencing. Quitting "cold turkey" is not an option. I follow the doctor's instructions for cutting back. It is no easy task. I begin to understand the level of determination it takes for addicts to say no to a pill-induced Nirvana. Nor is it an easy task to re-enter my former life.

I don't want to burden David with even more on his already overfull plate, so I struggle as best as I can to manage on my own and put on a happy face. Meal prep seems to take hours because of my need for frequent rests. I bless the "heat and eat" meals that land on our doorstop. Until I can drive again, I rely on friends to ferry me to appointments.

By March, I feel compelled to return to work at our business, even for a few hours a week. I continue IV-C treatments and Helixor injections, which help with healing but use up precious time and money. My treatment protocol is a serious drain on David's bank account. Ever grateful for that support, I don't want to feel like a burden any longer than necessary.

Every three months I re-visit Cross for CT scans, blood work, and a doctor's exam. Tense until I get the results, I always breathe a sigh of relief each time I am told everything is clear. Just entering the building is emotionally draining— too many bad memories!

While I am healing physically, I find myself searching for the gifts that cancer is supposed to bring. They seem to be a long time in coming. I believe that much of it has been about learning to receive – being willing to ask for and accept help just because I need it. I take the help most gratefully, yet reluctantly. Sometimes I doubt whether I am a worthy recipient.

Most of all, I am grateful for the feel of sun on my face and the joy of being alive.

Chapter 10

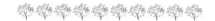

Every story I create, creates me. I write to create myself.   Octavia E. Butler

In August of 2012, the unthinkable happens. The latest scan reveals that my cancer has come back in the same spot. Smaller than the first lesion, it is there, nonetheless. To say I am devastated is an understatement at best. I was so sure that I had learned whatever lessons cancer had come to teach me. What have I missed? I feel like such a failure. Now what? In the face of this news, the last thing I want to do is tell anyone.

I have been on so many prayer lists, had so much support from so many people. I don't feel worthy of asking for more support – more help. Of course, as soon as I tune into this feeling of unworthiness, I realize that cancer still has something to teach me – I had learned during the first round about how to receive, but a vital piece of my growth is still missing.

Am I really worthy of receiving simply because I exist?

With surgery as the only option now that chemo and radiation have failed, my oncologist refers me to his choice of surgeon – a delightful young woman, Dr. Erica Haase, with a kind and compassionate nature. She carefully walks me through the steps of what will happen next and what the outcome will be – the dreaded colostomy bag.

Based on the way I have been feeling internally, I know that if I desire any quality of life, surgery is my only hope. Resigned and no longer so terrified about this path, I say yes. The surgery is scheduled for the end of September.

I visit Dr. DeNault for his pre-surgery protocol – some intense Vitamin B, C, and mineral therapy intravenously to build my immune system and promote healing after surgery.

A weekend retreat to Jasper helps us prepare mentally, emotionally, and spiritually. Not surprisingly, my family and friends rally round once again. I lean on their strength and grit, for I seem to have little of my own. I want to be as prepared as I can be in facing this step. I am equally determined to seek whatever answers I need to free me from lingering fears of a future bout of cancer.

Lorene, a dear friend, sends me a link to the website of a hypnotherapist, Dr. Francisco Valenzuela, whose specialty is working with oncology clients. As I read his web content, I feel an instant connection. I phone immediately for an appointment. Miraculously, he calls back on his day off and offers a spot the day before my surgery.

Our first meeting is like a breath of the freshest air. We chat for two hours. He projects such a ray of hope for my ultimate healing. His wife, Matilde, a psychologist, had recovered from two bouts of cancer herself. His assurance that the three of us will work as a team to discover the root cause of my disease is a balm to my spirit. I vow to return once I am healed enough from the surgery.

Recovery from surgery is easier in some ways, yet more difficult in others. I soon discover that a patient in a regular hospital is treated quite differently from patients residing at the cancer clinic. Don't get me wrong, I have had very caring and dedicated staff at both places. But the stretch to our health care system shows the difference in care levels. Whether you feel capable of managing after surgery or not, the quicker they can send you home, the happier they are. (Maybe that's why the food is so bad in hospital!)

Physically, I lose body parts and have been re-engineered in a way that is hard to deal with emotionally. They removed my rectum along with the cancer, re-routed my large intestine and pulled a piece of my colon through a hole in my abdomen, just to the left of my navel. That end piece was formed into what's called a "stoma" – my new asshole.

The ostomy nurses teach me how to deal with the bag that will be my companion for the rest of my life. It's yucky and messy, and I hate it. It gives new meaning to the phrase, "Get your poop in a group." Oh, goody. Not only will I have it in a group, it's in a very visible bag for easy access!

Worse news though, is that my somewhat functioning vagina has also been sacrificed on the healing altar. Crap! Nothing prepares me for this blow.

I go home with lots of soreness and more stairs to climb. The health care nurse visits as often as needed to check my incisions and answer my questions regarding stoma care. I feel weak, damaged, and vulnerable.

My Journal
October 2012

As soon as I can drive safely and sit somewhat comfortably for an hour, I start my weekly sessions with Dr. Valenzuela. My work with him gradually leads me back to myself. I learn anew the importance of honoring and nurturing my inner child.

I now see that my attempt to fix others in my life has been a misplaced need to heal myself. I've been a lost girl who hasn't felt worthy of receiving nurturing and healing. Cancer intervened to shine the light on this behavior. While everyone in my life has given me what they could over the years, ultimately, I'm the one charged with providing the nurturing that I need.

As a child, I had been trained young to be of service – that I must put everyone else's needs before my own – that my worth as a human being is determined by the amount of my service. My needs are last in line. Because of that lifelong conditioning, it's been so easy to set myself aside and to allow others to set me aside in favor of their own needs.

I'm enjoying my work with Dr. Valenzuela. He is my catalyst for growth. He said yesterday that in fighting to find my new purpose in life, there will be no room for cancer cells to take hold again. My immune system will just get stronger and stronger so it can deal with any rogue cells, as it has already done throughout my life. Though I don't quite believe it yet, I cling to this lifeline.

After a few sessions, I have a revelation. Through sharing my history, I can pretty much pinpoint when the cancer started. It was after I left my second husband. I was so distraught, so enraged, and so exhausted from that breakup that my body was fertile ground for cancer to burrow in. Research has long validated the connection between stress and cancer. Though I had not realized it, my stress has been both huge and prolonged.

I now see that all the healing protocols I tried only provided a temporary fix. Unless I address the heart and soul of me and seek understanding, forgiveness, and healing within, healing will elude me. Through poetry and art, I pour out my anger, my misery, and my grief. I start to feel stronger.

While I grow stronger physically and emotionally, the aftermath of surgery signals the death of David's and my faltering relationship of five years. It seems a tragedy that we won't get the fairy tale "happily ever after" ending. As much as we care for one another, David and I are too different to be able to build a life together. Everything we each dreamed of is never going to happen while we stay together.

Since we had vowed early in our relationship that neither of us would settle for less than the best, it has become too painful to continue as a couple. He has given his all to help me through my worst. Now it's up to me to forge my new path – alone.

It's the end of January 2013. I begin to look for work and a place to live. I pick the first job that comes along – a sales job in the sign business with enough base salary to cover my expenses. David helps with new furniture and the move. I spend my 63rd birthday in my new apartment. Month by month, it's a time of frantic activity to generate enough income to keep me solvent.

The bright spot of the year occurs on July 27th – the day my Trevor marries his lovely Kristina. She asks if I want to say something at the reception. Well, no one has ever had to ask me twice to speak!

At the podium I get a bit choked up as I realize how profoundly grateful I am to be alive to witness such a wonderful occasion. My first dance ever with my son after dinner is better than icing on a wedding cake – a sweet memory I will treasure forever.

As the rest of the year unfolds, although my job is providing for my financial needs, it takes its toll on my physical, mental, and emotional well-being. I begin to realize that I have seriously underestimated the time my body needs to fully recover. I stick it out as long as I can, quit and then spend the last six weeks of the year resting, reflecting, and meditating about the kind of life I want to create next.

Though I feel quite guilty at first for not going to work like everyone else, employment insurance buys me some time. I soon relax into a daily routine that works much better for me. A picture of my ideal life begins to take shape. The structure of it involves me working from home.

It still bothers me that after all I had been through since my near-death experience in 2007, that I still have not tapped into a new purpose.

Gradually though, I begin to feel little nudges about telling my story to groups – more platform-type speaking than workshops. But I don't feel ready to share that much about an experience that is still so raw. It is time to immerse myself in my own internal process.

Chapter 11

*If it is bread that
you seek, You will
have bread.*

*If it is the soul
you seek, You will
find the soul.*

*If you understand this
secret,
You know you are that which you
seek.* **Rumi**

At the beginning of my cancer journey, I couldn't let go of the notion that I was responsible for creating my cancer. Since my early training in personal growth in 1974, I have come to believe that everything in life happens for a reason, and at the root of it is me. While most of the doctors and psychologists were quick to assure me that I had not created my cancer – it was just something that happened – nobody's fault - somehow it didn't ring true to me. I really wanted to believe them because I was terrified of the enormity of owning the full responsibility of the outcome.

It is Neale Donald Walsch's book, *Communion with God,* that throws me the next lifeline. I had not wanted to accept my role and responsibility as creator of my cancer because of the judgment I placed around that. Who in their right minds would subject themselves to such a horrific thing that would involve not only themselves but their loved ones?

But if I remove the "bad", the "wrong" part – in other words, eliminate the judgment; could it be that I had created the cancer for my highest good and the good of all concerned? Had I created the experience to help me grow in a way that would not have been possible any other way?

I feel and accept the *yes* at a soul-deep level. This knowing is as true as what I had experienced in my 2007 journey to the other side. Can it be that I have created all of it, the good, the bad, and the ugly. As I review all the significant events of my life, I know that I have created them all – some consciously, many unconsciously. One thing has led to another, which led to another. The perfection of it all is astounding!

Now you need to know that I certainly don't consider myself evolved enough to have been the "conscious" instigator of everything. I believe we come into our physical existence purposely forgetting who we really are and why we are here.

But in the higher realms of Self, I believe I needed the epiphanies from my death experience in 2007. The spiritual "full-blown ecstasy" I experienced seeded the ground and prepared me for the cataclysmic cancer adventure that was to follow. I needed that knowing and assurance of life everlasting – that there is a plan and that everything happens for our highest good – even if we don't know what that is at the time.

Being the quintessential Pollyanna, I knew in my heart at the beginning of the cancer road that there would be gifts. I had no idea what they would be nor did I know that it would take two rounds of the disease and the subsequent sacrifice of body parts to reveal them.

But the knowing and the gifts do come in their time. The first gift is feeling and understanding at a deep level that I am worthy to receive all the help, care, attention, and love I need just because I exist – I matter to the people in my life. I don't have to "do" anything to earn it – I just have to "be".

As a Child of Spirit, I matter. Nothing can or will ever take that love away. We are always surrounded by that love. Having that understanding penetrate my heart and warm my very core adds strength – helps me to rise like the Phoenix, from the ashes of my despair.

I think about the years of misery, where I had struggled so hard to measure up, to serve others well, to be regarded as a good person so I could earn the right to the love and attention that I sought. But it was never enough, and I feared I would never be enough. I am the one who pushed myself away from the Love that has always been there for me.

Back I dive into "Communion with God". His words are like a balm to my soul. While I heal physically, I pick up the book and either read from beginning to end, or just open it at random and seek whatever message there is for me.

As for finding meaning and purpose in my life, more understanding comes from my bookshelf. Books have always called to me. I had read many spiritual, self-help, and metaphysical books during my intense personal growth phase in my 20s.

The passages that cover life meaning and the discovery of what matters to a person cause some deep soul-searching. What meaning had I given to my life? Why do certain things matter to me, and others don't? Had I been born with a purpose – yet to be discovered, or am I supposed to figure it all out and create it while here?

As I mull this over, the events of my life spin through my head. Why I had chosen the paths I did, why I had developed certain of my talents, how I had used my skills and talents to contribute in a meaningful way.

All of it becomes so obvious to me now. From the second I was born; it has been perfect in the way it unfolded. I marvel at the beauty of the tapestry that is my life.

I can see that the task before me is to decide what matters to me now – what does life mean to me in the aftermath of all my adversity? My lengthy "dark night of the Soul" has proved fertile soil for the growth of new understandings and awakenings. It feels as if I have received the kiss of Life from the handsome prince – I am awakening to glorious possibilities.

I have proven my strength and resilience to myself. While always believing in the magnificence of others, perfect in all their humanness, now it is time to believe in my own magnificence.

Phoenix

©Sue Paulson

Burned to ashes
dust blown away,
I sit in emptiness.
Lost, searching, alone.

All that matters,
matters not, anymore.
I wait,
cry into the silence.
Mourn the old.
Time passes.

Pin feathers
of new wonderings
emerge.

Flickers of light
dance behind
closed eyelids.
Rose gold,
flames of violet
beckon me home.

My heart
opens to new feelings,
pink skin.
I breathe in life,
love, tenderness,
meaning.

I grow and grow to be
Me.
Phoenix Risen.
Awash in Ecstasy.

Now what will I do with this knowledge and wisdom? I believe part of my journey involves finishing the manuscript I had started after my near-death experience. There is a reason it wasn't finished before – because I hadn't yet lived the rest of the story.

In January of 2014, my buddy, Pam invites me to a personal growth evening. Other than to enjoy it with her, I have no idea why I'm here. In my brief sharing with the group, I discover that what I know and what I have experienced means something to those listening. The sum of my experiences is not mine to keep, they are mine to share –others who are struggling to grow need to hear what I know.

Two months later, I attend a spiritual gathering conducted by a guy from Winnipeg called Dan King. This young man channels Spirit with a "no holds barred" approach to real life. His information is familiar, refreshing, and very reassuring. I have no idea what my connection to him is, but his return to Edmonton six weeks later at the behest of Spirit has me focusing more strongly on possibilities for my future work.

Growth has always meant as much to me as breathing. I am beginning to realize that my own meaning and purpose has always come from sharing what I know that could help others with their own growth and understanding. Maybe I just need to re-invent much of what I have already taught for so many years – only come from an entirely new perspective.

Serendipity is a wonderful thing. In March, a "chance" meeting with Suzanne Harris. A writing coach and friend, Suzanne tells me about her adventures of taking writers on a yearly retreat to Greece.

That gets my attention! As I ask her for more details, I can see myself there. I don't know how I will afford it, but somehow, I know I will be on that plane in September. My goal while there - finish my book. Soon after I pay my deposit, paid work pours in my door to make that dream a reality.

On September 15, our little band of writers lands in Athens.

We set out almost immediately to check out the sights. Our second day there, we tread the ancient roads to the Acropolis.

As I gaze down into the amphitheater on our way to the Parthenon, I burst into tears and sob uncontrollably. The ancient stage calls to me as if I have been there before – not only there, but on that stage.

I can't seem to get enough of the sights, the sounds, and the tastes of this wonderful place. Our hotel has a rooftop garden where we gather with wine at the end of the day. Our first glimpse of the Acropolis lit up at night is inspiring. Photo-op! I think I have posed for more pictures on this trip than I have ever done on any of my other travels.

Of course, there is also shopping for treasures and the quest for Greek food – Suzanne has her favorite places – we are happy to trot along and tuck into platefuls of dolmades, spanakopita, Greek salad, and whatever else catches our attention. Don't get me started about the homemade bread, and the olives, and dessert…sigh! Yes, I know – we are here to write – but a girl's gotta eat!

Our three days of sightseeing in Athens complete, we board the bus for the five-hour ride to Kardamyli – an enchanting little village surrounded by sea and hills that we will call home for the rest of our stay. The Mediterranean is never far from view as the bus traverses the switchback roads. I can't wait for a swim!

1978 was the first time I had been to this part of the world, though I hadn't visited Greece. I had fallen in love with the Mediterranean then, so I'm glad to be back.

The four of us split into pairs and share the two-bedroom suites in Antonia's Apartments. Stephanie, my roomie, and I have the magnificent seaside view from our spacious balcony. She graciously leaves me the biggest bedroom. Day or evening, it is a breathtaking vista. How will I ever get any writing done?

We soon find our daily rhythm - surreal days of trips up the hill to the market for breakfast and lunch fixings, time for musing and writing,afternoon swims and debriefs at night at a local eatery. We agree on this informal goal to eat our way through the village – though I am not sure our stay will be long enough! Each day I marvel that I am in such a special place. What a priceless gift I have given myself!

My manuscript has been housed in a series of electronic files that had accumulated over the course of seven years. My goal is to go home with a draft that has all the pieces in order. It seems like a mammoth, laborious task – one that I dread because there is little that is creative and so much that is tedious.

I struggle, but bit by bit most of my documents and journals turn into a more useful format. Unfortunately, I am left with about 16 documents that don't seem to fit anywhere. In disgust, I just number them and move everything to the end of the manuscript. I am pretty discouraged with the result and want to just trash it all. I imagine gathering all the documents and flinging them into the sea.

Disgruntled and sore from such a long sit, I walk up to the village for a change of scenery. When I get back to the courtyard of the apartments, I bump into Elias, our host. He and his mom, Mrs. Antonia run the business and look after us so well. Elias is a talented poet and philosopher. Sharing the stone steps, we have already had some heartfelt discussions about life.

He sees my distress and asks, "Mrs. Sue – what's the matter?"

I don't hesitate to tell him. "Have you ever been through something that was pretty horrific, started writing about it, and then thought, 'Oh who cares anyway – I lived through it and am on the other side of it. What does it matter, now?" I say.

His reply goes straight to the heart of it all. "Mrs. Sue, your story is not just your story – it belongs to us, too. It matters to us." His perspective is all it takes to settle me down.

My session the next day with Suzanne gets me back on track as she suggests a new starting point for the manuscript. I start to copy and paste. By the time I have 2000 words transferred into the newest draft, I am happy with my progress and keen to finish once I get home.

Because I have extended my stay beyond the formal retreat, I still have a few days to absorb the ambiance. Am I ever glad of the extra time! With my writing goal achieved, these days give me time to visit any sights I have missed and time to re-visit favorite spots. I spend more than a few minutes envisioning staying forever.

It is a tearful departure. Mrs. Antonia gives me a jasmine flower for my hair and wishes me well. I give Elias a few pages of my poetry – some that I have written while here and some older ones I think he will enjoy. He autographs one of his poetry books for me. Not all of it is in English, so I will need to brush up on my Greek!

More pictures and more tears as the bus winds its way up the mountain and gives me my last glimpse of Kardamyli. I vow to come back one day for another dip in the sea.

After a week of re-grouping at home, I contact Dan King for a phone session. Before my trip, I had decided to book a consultation upon my return from Greece.

With Dan as the conduit, Spirit has a lot to say about my trip to Greece and the two lifetimes I had lived there in the past – one male and one female. My resonance with and tears at the amphitheater had signaled the upcoming reality of being on stage again. I am told that as a Greek woman, I had lived not far from Kardamyli and swum in that same spot.

The information Dan gives is so valuable that I take copious notes. His was not the first session I had ever had with Spirit, but this one is timely and extremely powerful. It feels wonderful to be so at home in the presence of Spirit. We talk about my book – it's important that I finish it.

Chapter 12

Here is a test to find whether your mission on earth is finished: If you're still alive, it isn't.
Richard Bach, "Illusions"

2015

I continue to have a clean bill of health. In 2014, with my oncologist's blessing, I stopped my regular visits to the cancer institute. I remember the relief and extreme sense of joy when I exited that building!

With that chapter of my life closed, I often reflect about the why's and what's of all that has transpired:

- When I knew that the power existed to heal myself from cancer, why couldn't I do it?

- Why did I choose to experience it all – the ravages of chemo and radiation, the sacrifice of surgery, the benefits of alternative therapies?

- What was the point of all that pain, all the losses, and all that suffering?

- What next? What will I do with the gifts that I've been given from those experiences?

Reflections

Cancer calls.
Will you use it to wake up to a new life,
Or
Will you use it to take you Home?
Regardless – there will be gifts.
Cancer is not the enemy but a
ferocious friend that invites us
to search the deepest parts of ourselves
For ultimate healing.

It's a grand miracle, this playground we call life on earth.

The more conscious I become of how we're all connected, the more delight I can take in what I experience. I've begun to understand that what matters to me and what I choose to do about it is what gives meaning to my life. As I change and grow, so does my meaning.

A wise group of entities from the '70s who called themselves The Evergreens once said, "We are here to experience the experience of experiencing." Now that matters to me!

What is life now like for me? I view it as regeneration, not retirement. Life's daily struggles still exist, but they amuse me more than they annoy me. Any pity party I host bores me quickly and is soon over.

I'm more focused on drawing happiness from work, events, and the people in my life. I've learned that when I'm happy, it rubs off on others.

There's an old Zen saying:

"Before enlightenment, Chop wood,
Carry water.
After enlightenment,
Chop wood,
Carry water."

While I see the Light more clearly now and feel lighter every day, I still chop wood and carry water. The dust bunnies create a ruckus as they cavort under my bed. Paper messes, though fewer are still the bane of my existence.

My habit now is to focus more on serving my own needs first before turning my attention to serving others. When I'm stuck, rather than soldier on alone, more often I ask for help from others. I have surrounded myself with trusted professionals who work on this body that is no longer 18!

Even better, I have a growing group of like-minded friends of all ages who are there for me as I am for them.

George Bernard Shaw once said, "I want to be fully used up when I die." I echo that sentiment. I plan to wring as much joy as possible from this renewed life.

Out of my magnificent misery has come infinite peace and boundless joy. Out of adversity, I am blessed to experience ecstasy – full blown.

In the melodic symphony that is my life, I have before me another part to play before that final crescendo. Whether I show someone how to bend a spoon, invite others for Tea with Sue, write that book of fiction for my hoped-for grandchildren, or simply revel in the taste of a second piece of strawberry-rhubarb pie, it's all a magnificent adventure!

If there is one gift I can give you in parting, it is the gift of fully remembering, trusting, and experiencing your own magnificence. Each of us is truly magnificent in our own right. And guess what? It is safe to be as magnificent as you are. You came here with this magnificence, and you have it still – even if you don't acknowledge it or don't do anything with it. It is a wondrous part of every fiber of your being.

My friend, what will you do with your magnificence in the face of this precious gift of life? There is no right or wrong in what you choose – only consequences of those choices. Even if the outcomes of your choices don't please you, guess what? In all your magnificence, you can choose again, choose differently.

Just don't be surprised along the way if your Higher Self throws a little something extra into the mix, just to make you and your life even more magnificent! Until we meet again,

Be Who You Are

Be Your Magnificence

We Are All One!

Afterword

It's 2023 – 16 years after near-death, 12 years after the cancer diagnosis, and 8 years since this book was first published. So much has happened for me! Here I am at 73 with an ever-growing delight in my life and the lives around me. Oh, and five years ago, I was gifted with twin granddaughters!

Professionally, a year after Magnificent Misery was launched, this Voice (you know that Voice) said, "Sue, you're not done writing about cancer." We argued; I ignored it, but the Voice won. It won because I saw the increasing stats of people getting cancer, despite the billions of dollars being spent on the problem.

It seemed time to write more, so I began The Healing Call of Cancer - scheduled for launch in 2024. While there is some of me and my story in the new book, mostly it's how-to guide and a support for cancer sufferers, survivors, and their families.

Following are the opening pages of *The Healing Call of Cancer*.

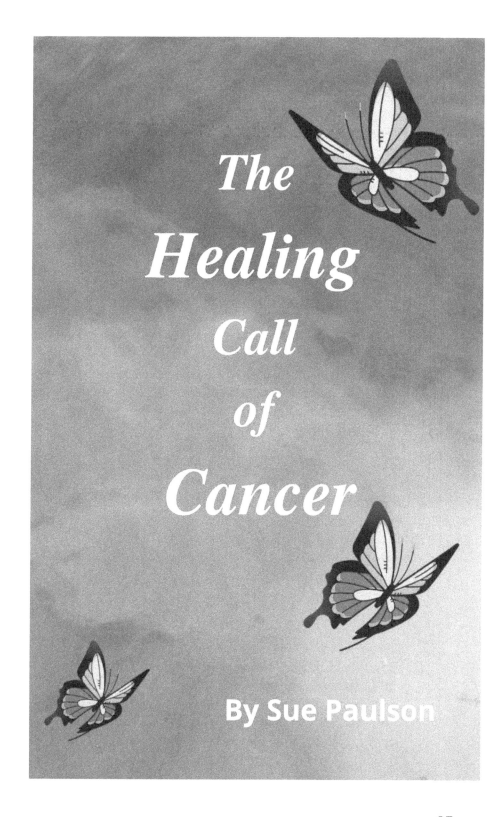

The

Healing

Call

of

Cancer

By Sue Paulson

"The Offering

The goal of this book is to support cancer sufferers as they face one of life's most challenging journeys. Not only have I survived cancer twice, but I have thrived for the past 11 years. I am not a medical professional or a researcher. The words I have written are from the perspective of a fellow sufferer.

As I share what I lived, what I discovered, and what I learned, my fondest wish is that you, my readers, will find lifelines, tools, and/or rays of hope to assist you on this path, not only through cancer but to a life beyond.

Just as other humans do, I have biases for and against certain things. For example:
I look for good in everything. I believe there are gifts in and even from the darkest of life's moments. Some call me the quintessential Pollyanna. I confess, that's me.

I do not believe that cancer just happens randomly to people – there is a reason – a good reason that you got it, and I got it. It didn't come from outside our bodies like an enemy invader. It has grown within our bodies as a signal that all is not well.

I believe that cancer has much to teach us about ourselves, our lives, and about the world we live in. It may take time to figure out why you and cancer became acquainted.

The way I chose to heal is not the only way. If something I say doesn't resonate with you, set it aside and keep searching for what could work for you. There are many books, internet articles and the experiences of others that can help you. I honor each of you in your quest for life beyond cancer."

Sue Paulson

Cancer & Me

This cancer has hollowed me out.
Stripped me of the bones of everything I ever
knew, was, or thought I could be.

Who am I now,
with the specter of death
hovering so near?

I seek my old self
and find but echoes
of a life I believed
was well-lived.

How do I proceed?

Can I create anew,
or will life's uncertainty
stop me in my tracks?
Will Fear be the victor?

©*Sue Paulson*

The Healing Call of Cancer - Excerpt

Reflections

Cancer calls.
Will you use it to wake up to a new life,
Or
Will you use it to take you Home?
Regardless – there will be gifts.
Cancer is not the enemy but a
ferocious friend that invites us
to search the deepest parts of ourselves
For ultimate healing.

Cancer has called you. Here you are, face to face.
The great unknown beckons – to what you don't yet
know. But you have been here before – on the precipice
of some other kind of adversity. Remember how you
were stronger than all those other adversities? You are
stronger now – stronger than this terror, and stronger
than this cancer. I know that you are strong enough to
go head-to-head with this cancer.

Likely this cancer feels like the enemy – the enemy that
could kill you. No wonder you're scared! In 2011, I
stood in the same spot as you when cancer called; I felt
the same terror. You need to know you are not alone.

Even though I will share bits of my story in these pages,
so you understand where I'm coming from, this book is
about You. Take what feels right – what resonates with
you – and leave the rest. I don't have a "cure". I don't
have The Answer. What I have are thoughts,
experiences, suggestions, and guidance that may help
you heal.

This book is divided into three distinct parts: body, mind, and spirit. I've come to understand that while the initial focus to eradicate cancer cells must be centered on the physical body, full healing comes from an additional intense focus on the mind and the spirit. It will take the holy trinity of YOU to not only survive cancer, but to thrive beyond it.

Now let's entertain the possibility that cancer has arrived in your life to become your teacher, your catalyst – your wake-up call. Like it or not, life is like that – it often tests us first – the learning comes later. For some of you, it's an opportunity to heal all of you so you can live life more fully than ever before. For others, it's the path to take that final journey Home.

Let's face it, our physical bodies are going to die of something, right? While we never know what will take us out and when that will happen, right now you are faced with that possibility. Since you can't know for sure whether you will live through or die from this cancer, you might as well opt for living through it. For whatever time any of us has left, it is possible that cancer will provide you an opportunity to learn to live the most joyful life possible while you're still here.

Regardless of your ultimate destination, this is a complex journey. Like exploring the facets of a diamond, you will be called to examine every surface of your physical, mental, emotional, and spiritual being. As with any hero's quest, you have some inherent power tools to support you on your journey:

Courage
Determination
Faith
Hope

Courage: In the face of fear, we can call upon our reserves of courage – we can even lean on others and borrow their courage. At times you will feel vulnerable. That's good. According to Brene Brown, there is no courage without vulnerability.

Determination: Humans are hard-wired to overcome adversity. When the going gets rough, we dig a little deeper for the energy to keep going.

Faith: Faith can move mountains. If you are a religious or spiritual person, your faith in a higher power is a mighty tool. Even if you are not part of a religion, you still have your faith in you to draw on, plus you have all the faith of your loved ones at your disposal.

Hope: Hope is defined as a feeling of trust – a feeling of expectation and desire for certain things to happen. When we build and maintain our hope for the best outcome, it sustains us through the darkest of times.

While none of these power tools can be seen or scientifically measured, collectively they make you tougher than any cancer. When you combine them with whatever treatment protocol you choose, you have the best chance of moving beyond cancer.

Available Spring of 2024

Meet the Sensational Sue Paulson!

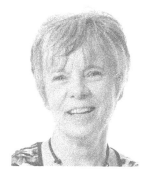

Despite her knocking knees, Sue got her first audience applause at age 10 after reciting a poem at church. Drawn to the front of the room, she started teaching a personal growth program in her late 20s. By 34, she was developing and conducting corporate workshops. At 42, she traveled Alberta as a paid speaker with topics such as stress reduction, conflict resolution, and team development.

A self-taught educator, Sue began the first of her 15 years of part time teaching at MacEwan University. Her topics - business writing, public speaking, and study skills.

In 1999 she published her first best-selling book, *Tips & Tools for Student Success.* It was followed in 2003 by her award-winning *Tips & Tools to Speak with Confidence.*

For her 50th birthday, Sue successfully challenged herself to perform 5 minutes of stand-up comedy on Amateur Night at Yuk Yuk's.

Thriving since her near-death experience in 2007 and bouts of cancer in 2011 and 2012, Sue published her memoir about those experiences, *Magnificent Misery – From Adversity to Ecstasy* in 2015. She has since launched her free app, The Magnificence Mentor.

Want more from Sue? Download her free App, The Magnificence Mentor from Google Play or the Apple store.
https://www.yourmagnificencementor.com

Then, sign up as a free member to unlock extra content, including
- Tea with Sue
  104 videos with Sue sharing thoughts about what life is teaching her.
- Magnificence Moments
  Short Videos to help you remove blocks and unlock your magnificence.
- Frivolishous Fridays
  Video Clips with Sue enjoying life and encouraging you to do the same.
- Healing Call of Cancer
  Videos designed to provide cancer sufferers and their families with information and hope
- Heaven on Earth
  Sue's thoughts about ways to create heaven, right here, right now.

To Book Sue as Your Next Inspirational Speaker, visit her website:
https://www.yourmagnificencementor.com

or e-mail her: sue@yourmagnificencementor.com

Her Topics Include:
- The Magnificence Matrix
- The Healing Call of Cancer
- Creating Your Brand of Heaven on Earth
- Pathways to Magnificence
- Sharing Stories – Leaving Legacies

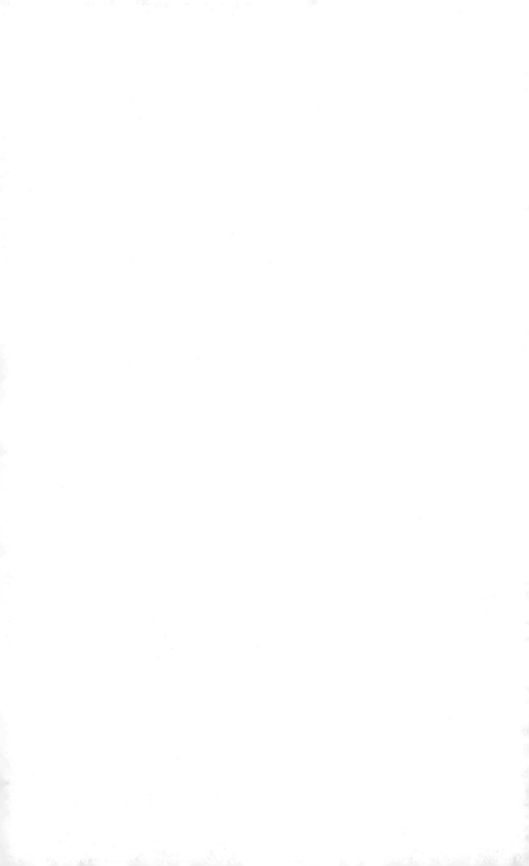